PRAISE FOR *MASTER*

"Cate Stillman is the leading voice in cutting-edge, evolutionary Ayurveda. This book is a take on ancient Five Element Theory, unlike anything I've ever read (but always secretly wanted). Ayurveda is a core wisdom that *must* evolve alongside us, and no one gets the need to modernize Ayurveda more than Cate. Read this book if you want all the sacredness of the ancient synthesized by the great mind of this woman. Read it if you want to add jet fuel to your life dreams."

KATIE SILCOX
New York Times bestselling author of *Healthy, Happy, Sexy*
and founder of The Shakti School for Women

"For more than 25 years, I've known Cate Stillman to live a life aligned to global positive impact and freedom. With *Master of You*, she innovates on ancient human wisdom to wake each and every one of us up to the core of our unique life and personal purpose. You'll get clarity on what you are here to do with your life, how to take immediate action, and enjoy the ride."

JIMMY CHIN
Academy Award® winner in Best
Documentary for *Free Solo* (2018)

"*Master of You* is masterful map to help you actualize your potential in the world. Cate Stillman guides you to awaken the five elements of Ayurveda to attune your ambition into action, become competent in your unique power, and design your life to result in the vitality and success you want to experience."

ELENA BROWER
author of *Practice You*

"In *Master of You*, Cate Stillman has manifested a bold blueprint for living your best life. Drawing from the holistic wisdom of yoga and Ayurveda, she gives readers a clear path to achieving things great and small. This book provides a proven and methodical way to reflect on your past, rewrite your personal history, and build a grand vision for your future—to show the world (and yourself) who you are capable of becoming."

YOGARUPA ROD STRYKER
author of *The Four Desires*, founder of ParaYoga, and creator
of the meditation and yoga nidra app Sanctuary

"Cate Stillman digs deep into ancient wisdom and modern practice to synthesize a marvelous and engaging journey to a better you. *Master of You* is the ultimate antidote to rampant narcissism haunting every aspect of our lives. She asks you to find your superpower, recognize the rhythms and cycles in your life, and tune in. She provides a path to purpose through caring for others. Read it—your friends, family, and coworkers will thank you!"

RICHARD E. BOYATZIS
professor at Case Western Reserve University and
coauthor of the international bestseller *Primal Leadership*
and the new book *Helping People Change*

"Ayurveda is clear: to be a Master of You, you must first pull back life's bow, hold it perfectly still, and then release yourself into the world from this calm and powerful place of heightened awareness."

DR. JOHN DOUILLARD, DC, CAP
founder of LifeSpa.com

"*Master of You* is like having a skilled, compassionate coach take your hand and direct you to live your best life. Cate Stillman's expertise and enthusiasm shine through every page. Using the power of the five elements, you will learn how to uplevel your health and time with joy."

HEATHERASH AMARA
author of *Warrior Goddess Training*, *Warrior Goddess Wisdom*, and *The Warrior Heart Practice*

"*Master of You* is a user-friendly life guide. This book offers a no-nonsense approach to knowing what you want, and making it happen. It is clear that Cate Stillman's decades of working and living in the modern world have arrived at a clear methodology for improving quality of life and setting the stage for self-evolution. This book is also an excellent guide for motivation for those on the spiritual path."

KATE O'DONNELL
author of *The Everyday Ayurveda Guide to Self-Care*
and *The Everyday Ayurveda Cookbook*

"Cate artfully adapts Ayurveda for modern times to help us calm and reinvigorate our distracted minds and bodies. *Master of You* is a guide to awaken a new 'you' through newfound purpose, giving you the power to become the master of your new destiny."

BRIAN SOLIS
author of *Lifescale: How to Live a More Creative, Productive, and Happy Life*

"A practical and compelling case to heed ancient wisdom in modern times to enrich your life and the lives of those around you."

PAUL JARVIS
author of *Company of One*

"Cate poses a provocative question—*Do you dare to dream big?*—and then proceeds to brilliantly map out a manifestation process through Five Element Theory. Cate is a master at taking esoteric Ayurveda and yoga philosophy and grounding it into our lives with clarity and relevance."

MARC HOLZMAN
renowned yoga teacher and Ayurveda practitioner

MASTER OF YOU

ALSO BY CATE STILLMAN

Body Thrive: Uplevel Your Body & Your Life with 10 Habits from Ayurveda and Yoga

Good Morning Yogis, Big and Small

MASTER OF

YOU

A Five-Point System to
Synchronize Your Body, Your Home, and Your Time with Your Ambition

CATE STILLMAN

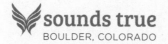

sounds true
BOULDER, COLORADO

Sounds True
Boulder, CO 80306

Published 2020

Cover design by Rachael Murray
Book design by Beth Skelley
Illustrations by Kara Fellows

Printed in Canada

Library of Congress Cataloging-in-Publication Data

Names: Stillman, Cate, author.
Title: Master of you : a five-point system to synchronize your body, your
    home, and your time with your ambition / Cate Stillman.
Description: Louisville, CO : Sounds True, Inc., 2020. |
    Includes bibliographical references and index.
Identifiers: LCCN 2019027902 (print) | LCCN 2019027903 (ebook) |
    ISBN 9781683642619 (paperback) | ISBN 9781683643166 (ebook)
Subjects: LCSH: Self-actualization (Psychology) | Yoga. | Medicine, Ayurvedic.
Classification: LCC BF637.S4 S824 2020 (print) | LCC BF637.S4 (ebook) |
    DDC 615.5/38—dc23
LC record available at https://lccn.loc.gov/2019027902
LC ebook record available at https://lccn.loc.gov/2019027903

10 9 8 7 6 5 4 3 2 1

To our collective human ancestors, who developed and refined the language of the elements so we can all unlock the powers within to live our best lives possible. And to the posse at Yogahealer.com, who cocreated the Master of You system with me.

The story of the human race is the story of men and women selling themselves short.

—Abraham Maslow, *Road Signs for Success*

Ayurveda recommends integrating your "being" into your "doing," so that your life is your "practice."

—Sebastian Pole, *Discovering the True You with Ayurveda*

You have to master yourself.

—My cab driver in Atlanta on June 13, 2019

CONTENTS

INTRODUCTION:
WHO COULD YOU BECOME NEXT?

What are your deeper ambitions?

I'm curious.

I'm curious about what you would do with your time if you were deeply rested, resilient, focused on your next creative desires, and had time to heed the deeper callings of your life.

I'm curious enough to have updated ancient human wisdom into an accessible system to help you activate and achieve your potential in the most honest and true way. I'm sensible enough to know that first, before heeding your deeper calling, you might need to improve your energy, resilience, desire, and relationship with time to take back control of your life.

So, we'll begin from where you are right now.

Right now, we are at a beginning together.

What do you want your life and yourself to be like next?

What path are you steering yourself toward?

What target are you aiming for?

If you could develop yourself into the person you want to become next, what is that person like?

What can she do?

What if you met your present realities, challenges, and opportunities facing forward, rooted from within, activating support from all around you? What if you could keep designing for and actualizing the life beyond your current wildest dreams? Who could you become?

Master of You is an invitation to heed the beckoning of your soul. Like our ancestors did, you can empower yourself with the sheer, raw, intuitive forces of the five elements of Ayurveda. Space (also as known as ether) element is the unknown in front of you; earth element is beneath your feet and in the rhythms pulsing through your veins; fire element lights your path, showing you the way forward and sparking passion to endure; air element is the wind power to orient you to the field of time in hours to decades ahead; and water element teaches you surrender, humility, and flow. In *Master of You*, you will befriend the elements as you activate your hero's or heroine's journey through your deeper dreams and into your unique creative potential, your *dharma*.

This journey of your becoming is reflected in the golden spiral. Also known as the golden ratio, the golden spiral is a pattern that occurs everywhere in nature, from galaxies to plants to your body. A golden spiral is created when infinite expansion spirals from a starting point and extends into the unknown. The cyclical iterations of expansion and contraction that unveil our innate intelligence and universal power also constitute a golden spiral. The Master of You program rides the evolutionary current—the golden spiral of you—from right here, right now into the future, and we'll reflect on this expansion into your potential on the journey ahead. In traversing the spiral, you'll ride the momentum of your learnings and your accomplishments thus far to fuel your next purpose. Throughout this process, I'll guide you through synchronizing your home, your body, your vision, and your time so you can experience a life of flow and integrity in fulfilling your ambition.

True ambition and self-leadership challenge us to be better, to transform. Bob Anderson and William Adams, authors of *Mastering Leadership*, wrote, "Transformation is an acquired taste—not for the faint of heart. However, significant culture shifts and performance require it. That's the deal."[1]

I want to recognize you for investing in your own transformation by picking up this book. Your attention is your most valuable currency, and you are your most valuable investment. We are smack-dab in a time labeled the *attention economy* and the *experience economy*. Together these terms recognize that we value, above all else, directing our attention to experiences. The highest rung on the ladder of experiences—the best use of our attention—is meaningful, transformational experiences. You want to "do you" better. We also want to "do us" better, to improve our relationships. We want purposeful lives, resilient bodies, inspiring homes, substantial relationships, and innovative projects. Living your life aligned to your purpose and potential is the transformation, and it is a process. *Master of You* provides an organized system, a sequence, that leads to self-mastery with your dharma—your bigger purpose—via the five elements.

HEEDING THE CALL

But first, as your guide, I'll share how heeding the call of ambition unfolded for me. During a summer in high school working on a volunteer wilderness trail crew under the tutelage of two environmental thought leaders, I picked up their worldview of looking for solutions to global problems. I saw solvable problems swirling around the health of the planet. This motivated me and a friend to form Students Concerned About Tomorrow (SCAT), an activist club focused on social diversity and ecological awareness. We quickly gave SCAT a platform and grew it into a small army for progressive initiatives.

In college, my curiosities centered on the intergenerational economics of climate change policy, which led to my working in Washington, DC, to reduce greenhouse gas emissions globally. Frustrated by policies that police unconscious and greedy behaviors to no avail, I turned my attention to helping humans become healthier, more vibrant, aware, awake, and ecologically connected beings.

This thread led me to the ancient wisdom of yoga and Ayurveda—the paths of enlightenment and radiant longevity—some of the oldest life-hacking systems iteratively tested and consistently practiced over millennia. And personally, I wanted to heal *myself* of increasingly chronic symptoms, including acne, allergies, excess body weight, negative self-talk, body judgment, constipation, migraines, and fibrocystic breasts.

By the turn of the century's dotcom bust, I was an Ayurvedic practitioner and professional yoga teacher. Over time, I built my company, Yogahealer.com, into a hub of innovative global course communities revolving around Ayurveda, dharma, detox, and health-coach training. I cultivated a knack for creating innovative curricula that reveal the hidden power of these ancient wisdom traditions for modern people. Close to two decades later, Yogahealer.com is still evolving and growing, with much of the recent interest focusing on dharma, or living your life on purpose, and leadership, which brings us to *Master of You*.

WHY YOU WANT TO MASTER THE FIVE ELEMENTS

In this age of digital distraction, as a global culture, we're struggling with our focus, creativity, anxiety, productivity, and personal purpose. Habituated to electronic devices, as a society we're overscheduled, overwhelmed, overfed, and under-rested. We've lost our sixth sense, which helped us navigate life according to our personal purpose, and sacrificed our health along with it. Yet, all-encompassing solutions to realigning our intrinsically and uniquely creative ambitions *lie within the five elements*.

Our human ancestors were so profoundly dependent upon and connected to the natural environment that they fundamentally communicated in terms of elements. Across cultures human thought, language, and conceptual understanding of who we are and how we came to be here developed from the elements: space, earth, fire, air, and water. In the first peoples' mythic stories, the elements are the building blocks of the universe and hold intrinsic powers that can be used to solve challenges and shape futures. Most of our ancestors naturally used a five-element system to heal disease, to thrive, and to awaken their personal and collective powers. For example, rather than press a button on an induction cooktop, our ancestors generated a spark with flint and steel. They tactilely and intrinsically understood the relationship between friction, spark, fuel, heat, light, and transformation—just in brewing a morning beverage. Disconnected from the elements in modern times, we sacrifice that innate wisdom; with it, we relinquish personal power, health, creativity, and the focus needed to live the life of our potential.

The five-element theory from Ayurveda is especially sophisticated and honed toward evolving yourself as an embodied spirit with purpose.

Ayurveda—a holistic, spiritual science of healing—was developed in India, along with yoga, more than 3,000 years ago. Ayurveda and yoga together—as different sides of the same coin—reflect a time-tested, experiential learning, self-optimization system empowered by the local ecosystem, reliant on inner wisdom, and pointed toward a life of purpose and creative freedom.

Our local and global cultures, with increasing disruption by technology and decreasing connection to the elements, have unintentionally lost certain powers. For example, inexpensive goods have generated clutter, which erodes our ability to design a home environment in which we can thrive (space element). With light stimulation after dark, our body rhythms no longer have the power of the circadian rhythm for hormonal balance (earth element). Our mental clarity and focus (fire element) are decreasing year after year as our electronic devices distract our attention. With too-busy schedules, we lose command over our time (air element). Missing the mark on how we want to live our lives and feel in our bodies, we lose the experiences of compassion, empathy, and flow along with our integrity (water element).

Each element holds an essential power. For example, to be grounded means you access the powers of earth and water elements. You are relaxed, centered, available, and able to support yourself and others. As you delve into learning about the elements, you'll notice you might have cultivated certain elements at the expense of others, leading to an imbalance. For example, if you focus on setting and hitting ambitious goals in a timely manner (fire and air qualities), you might sacrifice flow, joy, and ease (water and space qualities). When you pursue it chronically, this pattern leads to stress and health issues. On the flip side, if you develop the powers of ease and joy at the expense of achievement, you might have trouble prioritizing what you must do to move your life forward. You might opt for the easy road and never make your destination, or you might miss your mark. Neglecting an element within you is like forgetting an essential ingredient in baking a cake: you won't get the outcome you want. Dynamic harmony is when you are intuitively aware and empowered by all five elements and accessing their diverse qualities simultaneously. This harmony generates a larger capacity for an awake, purposeful life beyond your wildest dreams.

Master of You reconnects you to the elements to design the future you want to experience. You become skillful in perceiving and directing the five elements within you, steering your actions toward your ambitions—daily, seasonally, annually, and through the stages of your life. Simultaneously, *Master of You* awakens your joy, ease, creativity, health, and relationships. Through developing your hidden powers of space, earth, fire, air, and water, you captain your life from your soul.

TRIED AND TRUE: THE MASTER OF YOU SYSTEM

My first book, *Body Thrive*, codified the key daily habits of yogis into a simple system: ten practices plus the behavioral science basics on how to actually evolve those practices into habits. *Body Thrive* readers and online course members found that they experienced a steady daily surplus of energy, more time in their days, and more ease. They saved money they hadn't realized they were wasting. Not only did many of them heal chronic health issues (immune system, weight, hormonal, and stress) but their relationships became healthier, their self-compassion increased along with their feelings of inner fulfillment, and their desires became smarter and healthier. They started to wake up an internal desire to do more and to do something worthy. They wanted the next level of curriculum for manifesting greater ambitions.

So, I began sharing the concepts that I was living, which focused on the fundamental creative powers of the five elements. I learned to elevate my living environments (space), my rooted resilience and strong immune integrity (earth), my vision and planning (fire), my time (air), and my flow state (water). I next codified a five-element life-design system and created an online course to share these tools. The result is in your hands—a distilled, yet complete version of the system in a book, tested and improved by course members over the years. Along the way, I applied this process again and again to Yogahealer.com, growing both a business team and a volunteer mentoring leadership community, and as a result, it has ranked in the top 2 percent of US women-owned businesses in terms of revenue.[2] I've also followed my dream of living in two countries—the United States and

Mexico—surfing, paddle boarding, skiing, biking, and being what my child calls a "stay-at-home" mom while regularly getting a good night's sleep and making home-cooked meals. The Master of You family-related tools have been tested by my daughter and husband, evolving our communications and ability to steer ourselves toward our individual and collective dreams together. I'm not exceptional, but I am diligent about living my life aligned. I'll show you how to live your life aligned too.

A SYSTEM TO GUIDE YOUR TRANSFORMATION INTO MASTERY

The Master of You system is a sequence of actions, a *krama*, to steer your life from your soul using the elements. The Sanskrit term *krama* refers to an efficient route to a goal—a systematic process of distilled, sequential actions that generate a desired result. (Note: krama is different from *karma*, another Sanskrit term that describes the relationship between an action and the effect of that action, or the principle of cause and effect.) If you "do" this book chapter by chapter, exercise by exercise, mindful of the process, you leverage your time and attention with a well-tested sequence. Reflections, practices, journaling, and exercises guide you through the elements. As you awaken and wield your elemental powers, you continually leverage what you have accomplished to open the gate to what is next.

As when you climb a ladder, you get a bigger and better view with each rung. Working the process of your own transformation paves the way to greater delights, inspired relationships, health, wealth, and the capacity to steer yourself toward new horizons. To evolve and to advance levels is to *uplevel*. Similar to when you play some video games, when you master one level, you unlock the next. The skills you learned at the previous level are tested with bigger challenges that develop new skills.

Part of the process is to meet the challenges that arise as evolutionary adventures, however surprising or awkward. This is the game of your life. You are choosing to stretch yourself toward grander horizons while rooted in resilience. Tests of your commitment will arise. I will guide you through the work—to be a person who embraces the challenge as the adventure—to gain new skills and adapt. You will become more whole, powerful, and embodied, earning competencies and receiving true rewards. You will become an inspiration and a unique asset to those who know you. If you trust the system *and your process*, you'll access the grace of your own becoming. You'll become a boon to others. I'll be with you all the way, element by element, as you develop the skills, tools, and ethos you need to become who you want to as you turn your strengths into superpowers.

Eventually, Master of You becomes more than a program or a course: the exercises, the values, and the mindset all become your ingrained operating system as you integrate them into your life. The elements become you and your powers. Through iterations, you evolve; you navigate your life increasingly capable, resilient, adaptable, and curious about your next possibilities. What's more, as you become master of your life, you serve your next potential. At some point, though, we naturally tire of putting forth effort from a self-limiting or egoic place and offer our personal purpose to a greater good, allowing the supreme source to power our efforts and guide our intuition—this is a yogic concept called *ishvara pranidhana*. This aligned action happens from a clear mind and an awake heart, allowing us to navigate the next transformation without second-guessing or doubt.

Although transformation might be an acquired taste, it is the foundation of the Master of You system and the key to a life of presence that consequently leads to a life beyond your present dreams and a you beyond your current self.

Through living and teaching this process, I've witnessed people transform their health, personal purpose, career, relationships, and wealth. I've seen people heal long-term autoimmune diseases, resolve rifts and build thriving relationships, double their annual income and finance their dream home, align their family's lifestyle to their unique vision, and most important of all align their lives to their own definition of success. People also work this process with their teams, families, colleagues, and friends to achieve collective goals.

FIND YOUR POWER IN THE ELEMENTS

Evolution speaks through desire. Desire fuels a life of purpose. Below you'll find a checklist that you can use to treasure hunt for your current desires. As you tick boxes, note the elements with the most check marks.

If you think your desires seem selfish or indulgent, go a few layers deeper with your whys. For example, "I want more money." When you ask the why behind wanting more money, it might become "I want to take more time away from work"; the why behind that might be "I want more time to raise my children," and one step further might be "I want to raise my children to be courageous humans who love life and respect our planet." Repeatedly asking "Why?" reveals the desires that are not selfish or indulgent.

DESIRES OF SPACE

◯ I want to live and work in inspired spaces.

◯ I want to design my spaces to support the habits I want.

◯ I want to save money by not buying extra stuff.

◯ I want to live in a clutter-free space and
get my family onboard with that.

◯ I want to surround myself only with possessions that
add value, meaning, and direction to my life.

DESIRES OF EARTH

◯ I want to rise and shine and have a surplus of energy in the day.

◯ I want to be deeply rested.

○ I want to feel nourished.

○ I want my bones to carry the right amount of
muscle and fat for this stage of my life.

○ I want to experience calm centeredness.

○ I want peak performance and deep rejuvenation
as a daily experience, supported by the rhythms
of my household and workplace.

○ I want to switch from living in a state of stress to living with ease.

○ I want to keep my body moving as I age.

○ I want to befriend my unique constitution to empower my life.

DESIRES OF FIRE

○ I want to fulfill my evolving ambitions.

○ I want to be a visionary for my unique life
and encourage others to do the same.

○ I want to build successful strategies to
make my vision into reality.

○ I want to help groups I'm part of—at work or
home—also envision, strategize, and plan.

○ I want to morph my critical issues into my success strategies.

○ I want to leverage my strengths and competencies.

○ I want to repeatedly expand beyond who I have already been.

○ I want to articulate goals and receive help, guidance, and collaboration in reaching them.

○ I want to effectively and efficiently set and hit strategic milestones.

○ I want to intentionally, proactively author my life and encourage others to do the same.

DESIRES OF AIR

○ I want to have a spacious calendar, where I do what I want, when I want, more of the time.

○ I want my daily schedule to nurture my body rhythms and reflect my core values.

○ I want to break big projects into achievable action steps, personally and professionally.

○ I want to organize my time so I can focus and work on what is most important.

○ I want to automate the specific habits that lead me to reach my target.

○ I want my annual, quarterly, weekly, and daily rhythm to tune in to my vision, and I want to align my actions with my calendar.

○ I want to get the support I need to accomplish my bigger goals.

DESIRES OF WATER

◯ I want to be a person of great integrity.

◯ I want to be compassionate with myself and others on the path of transformation.

◯ I want to act from my intuition and live from my inner rhythm.

◯ I want to assimilate my shortcomings and turn them into my future strengths.

◯ I want to experience flow—not rush—in my daily life.

◯ I want to respect my pace through the changing seasons and stages of life.

◯ I want to be financially fluent, fluid, and accumulating.

From the checklists above, you can now see clearly what you want mastery over in the next phase of your life and the related element or elements.

HOW TO "DO" THIS BOOK

Some books you read. Other books you do. *Master of You* is designed for learning by doing. The exercises in each chapter are essential for achieving results and realizing the power of this system. You can download worksheets and stream guided audios to help you *do* the exercises in the accompanying free workbook, available at masterofyou.us/workbook. With iterations of the krama, the sequential system, you gain mastery with the five elements.

In working this method with hundreds of people, I discovered it's best to start with your deepest desires. For this reason, in part 1 of this book I aim to awaken your dreams, bolster your ambition, and rustle up your potential. Through this self-study—what yogis call *svadyaya*, or knowledge of the self—the elements and their laws, previously hidden in plain view, become visible. In chapter 1, you'll unearth your dreams and sense of personal purpose. In chapter 2, you will learn the basics of the five-element operating system of Ayurveda—the building blocks of mastery—which contain the universal laws behind our everyday reality. In chapter 3, you'll practice the mindset, or ethos, that accelerates self-mastery.

Thus prepared, in part 2 you will develop the five elements within yourself. You'll assimilate the five elements into your day and access their powers. Chapter 4 focuses on space element, and there, you'll learn how to uplevel your living and working spaces to support your goals. In chapter 5, on earth element, you'll build physical resilience through refining your body rhythms. In chapter 6, on fire element, you'll clarify your three-year vision, build your strategy to get there, and specify your one-year milestones and action plan for the next season. In chapter 7, on air element, you'll put your action plan into motion and into your schedule, commanding your time like a boss. Through making your vision real, you will unearth buried issues and missing skills. In chapter 8, on water element, you'll break through the new obstacles that appear on the path to your purpose by developing intuitive wisdom and healing gaps of integrity within yourself.

If you do these exercises iteratively, you'll empower yourself and your life, element by element. It's not uncommon for people to invest considerable time in one element before proceeding. By putting in the effort and sticking with it, they gain the power of that element and are ready to go on to the next one. They leverage what they have accomplished, opening the gate to what is next.

As at the cellular level you become more whole, integrated, and powerful, you will reveal your next unique ambitions. The method metamorphoses you into the next phase of your growth. Like a child who outgrows their jeans, you will become a bigger, more capable, and more heartful human. You will become who you haven't yet been. I will repeatedly ask you, "Who do you want to become next?" In the process, you will recognize your own plasticity and see your future in chapters. As you master the five elements within yourself and in your life, you become a master of you who evolves into a leader of us.

This is where the Master of You program begins.

PART I

Overview and Groundwork

1

UNEARTH YOUR DEEPER DREAM TO AWAKEN YOUR AMBITION

Take a moment to complete this sentence: "I can't wait until _____."

You might first fill in the blank with your urgent wants and desires. Perhaps you can't wait until a certain project is complete or your work week is done. Perhaps you dream of how your life might be when an event or a phase of your life is behind you. If you keep asking the question, you'll uncover deeper dreams you might wish you had already escorted to fruition. Your deeper dreams are revealed through your big desires, and these indicate your true ambitions, which lead to your deeper purpose. Your deeper dreams might be buried, dormant, or at the top of your mind. Any way you slice it, you're in the right place. Escorting your deeper dreams or next ambitions to the surface, to the front and center of your life, is the focus of this chapter.

Naming, acknowledging, and noting your wants and desires is a step toward action. Aligned action is what propels dreams into reality. Yet, often deeper dreams are submerged in layers of frustration, regret, fear, doubt, skepticism, or depression. As modern life gets busier, dreams get buried in the everyday whirlwind (see Figure 1.1). Days can get packed with activities that don't line up with our desires or priorities. Global culture today is on this trajectory: fast paced; hyperstimulated; undernurtured; overfed; overwhelmed; and inundated with activities, mental input, and physical stuff to process and organize. Our culture threatens our ability and sensibility to align our daily rhythms with our deeper dreams, ultimately preventing us from generating a healthier, more meaningful, thriving future.

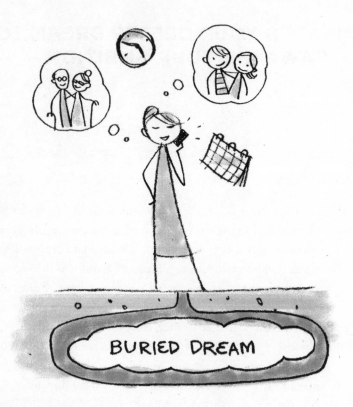

Figure 1.1 Buried dream

When you track and strategize your desires, your deeper dreams emerge. If you don't, you sacrifice your ability to create the life you want next. Over time, if you surrender to the whirlwind, you lose your connection to a possible future, to an even better version of yourself. Slowly and eventually, you can lose your faith in yourself, hope in your dreams, and belief in your potential and purpose. Self-doubt takes over. Therefore, with your dreams, much is at stake.

Ask yourself without self-denigration: Have you sacrificed your dreams to the whirlwind? Have you sacrificed your potential to the demands of the moment? If so, you're not alone. And you're reading this book, which will help you cultivate your power to design the next chapters of your life by showing you how to align your actions with your deeper dreams. Authorizing yourself to be self-authoring—to have the life you uniquely want and become the person you want to become—is part of the process. Activating your dreams leads to the desire to do something great, to live a life of greater purpose and impact, or at least to do something better than you have already done.

This self-determining creative power is *shakti*, which in Sanskrit, the language of yoga, is often translated as energy, power, or force. As you likely already know, yoga is the path of transformation, a union between your *self* and your ultimate potential. You can activate your creative power and transform or evolve your self. When you awaken this power already within—your *shakti*—you incrementally expand your potential for the possible in your life. (Note: Throughout this book, I'll use the words *power* and *shakti* interchangeably. I'll also exclusively use Sanskrit for terms that impart meaning diluted during their translation to English. The Sanskrit terms are defined in the glossary at the back of this book.)

Yogis believe humans contain levels of potentiality of which we are not ordinarily aware, and through specific habits and practices, we can activate these just as yeast activates flour and water to make dough rise. Shakti is the yeast that sets these new levels of potentiality into motion, allowing us to become conscious of them. Through cultivating your body, heart, mind, and relationships, you cultivate your shakti. In the process, you evolve your consciousness.

Developmental psychologists have identified stages of human consciousness. Within these stages, the three features that develop are: (1) cognition (what one is aware of), (2) values (what one considers most important), and (3) self-identity (what one identifies with).[1] This means that as we develop our awareness, what we're aware of transforms, what we value transforms, and who we are transforms. As we develop these features and advance our consciousness—what I refer to as *personal evolution*, *becoming*, and *identity evolution*—even greater desires, possibilities, and priorities emerge. Humans evolve from being self-serving to being community-serving and eventually to being life-serving. At higher levels of Buddhism and yoga, adepts vow to guide others into their spiritual potential and in the process are themselves transformed by serving.[2] Deeper levels of compassion and communication emerge on this universal trajectory of awakened, conscious, creative power—this is humanity's collective potential. Of course, you might have come to *Master of You* wanting a better personal reality—more time on your hands, more inspired and aligned people in your life, and more money in the bank. And that is a fine place to begin. Inevitably in the process your creative power will be systematically unlocked, and that will eventually lead to deeper purposes that serve the collective potential, ultimately resulting in your personal evolution.

This deep purpose, to heed the call of duty to your own divine ambition, is what the yogis call *dharma*. Medieval translations of dharma—such as duty, law, and right action, which can be connected to relationship, caste, and vocation—arise from dharma's ancient meaning in India. More ancient than that, the root of dharma is to uphold an obligation, or to support firmly. New-age words such as *soul purpose*, *life purpose*, and *raison d'etre* describe the modern interpretation of dharma. Clearly, dharma has levels of meaning. American Trappist monk Thomas Merton succinctly wrote this about dharma: "Every man has a vocation to *be* someone: but he must understand clearly that in order to fulfill this vocation, he can only be one person: himself."[3] In *Master of You*, you'll explore where heeding your call, your duty to participate fully in your life, is leading you next.

Dharma points you to a life only *you* can fulfill and uphold. With fewer cultural roles and rules than our ancestors had, our freedom to manifest our dharma is more accessible, unleashed, and tangible than ever. Dharma also points the way to your singular evolutionary impact as part of a living system, a larger cosmos. As Stephen Cope writes in *The Great Work of Your Life*, "Yogis believe that our greatest responsibility in life is to this inner possibility—this dharma—and they believe that every human being's duty is to utterly, fully, and completely embody his own idiosyncratic dharma."[4] Your duty to uphold your best potentiality, authentically and practically, while being part of transformational experiences that add connection and meaning to those whose lives you touch, is your dharma.

In my experience, your dharma, like a book, reveals itself in chapters, all of which stay true to your book's theme. If you've buried your desires and, with them, your powerful purpose, it's time to dig out that book, dust it off, and treat it like the exquisite jewel it is at the root of your being. You can learn how to listen to your dharma and to give it the gravitas it deserves in the conversation of what is next for you to become. In the process, you make the shift from feeling like life is on top of you to feeling that you are on top of life (see Figure 1.2).

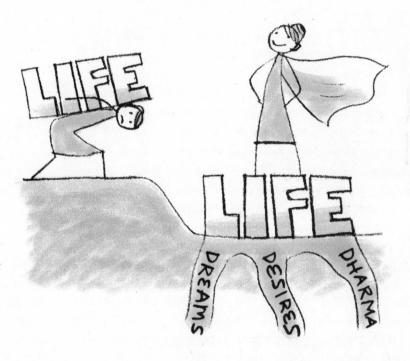

Figure 1.2 Are you on top of life?

Discover the Next Purpose Hidden in the Root of Your Self

Take a moment to pause. In your imagination, wipe the slate clean of today, tomorrow, and yesterday. It's blank and uncarved. To jump-start this conversation between you and your next purpose, set a timer for twenty minutes. Write or sketch in a journal using the sentence stems below. Trust your inner voice. Don't edit it.

1. "I can't wait until _____."

2. "Who I'd like to become next is _____."

3. "The next purpose hidden at the very root of my self might be _____."

Over the next week, read it in bed every night before you go to sleep, and then read it again every morning when you wake up. At these times of day *liminal thinking*—that is, thinking beyond your normal threshold or your patterned mind—is most active. As you read your words or look at your sketch, edit them to *true* your words like a bike mechanic trues the spokes of a wheel to remove the wobble, align the spokes, and optimize efficiency. You are awakening the creative agent in your life, an identity you'll develop through mastering yourself. In this self-mastery process, you will honor your root, reawakening desires to guide your future and to steer yourself on your path. ■

BIG PROBLEMS FOR THE HEART, THE MIND, AND THE BODY

Big problems arise when your daily life is off course. You might notice it in your gut or heart first. Then you'll notice it in your mind and then in the rest of your body. For example, you might not love the pace of your life. You sense your gut or heart sinking when you look at your calendar and feel like you have to go through the motions. As you go through the motions, your mind checks out, looking for distractions—coffee, sugar, weed, wine, an extra serving, social media or other sticky apps, online or brick-and-mortar shopping—any of which increases your whirlwind. If this downward cycle of disconnection continues, eventually your immune integrity—the unified field of your heart, mind, and body—follows suit into dis-integration, and a diagnosable mental or physical disease develops.

When the rhythm of your life is no longer in tune with circadian rhythm, you have a problem. The circadian rhythm—the twenty-four-hour cycle of all living beings—connects healthy body rhythms to healthy mind rhythms to healthy heart rhythms (both physically and metaphysically). Unfortunately, our culture is on fast forward without pause, out of rhythm. Perhaps there was a turn in your heart's desires, and you kept going straight. You might have ignored the desire to shift—*upshift* or *downshift*. Current culture is weak on winding down, reflection, and closure. Without reflection or tuning in, you can't recognize when a shift, a purpose-deep realignment in your life, is needed. Reflection is the part of a cycle that naturally realigns your inner desire to your outer life—your space, your time, your activities—into an even brighter future. Reflection asks you to re-collect your yearnings, your regrets, and even your skepticism.

UPDATE YOUR RECORDS

Your yearning and regret not only unlock the contemplative joy that comes from deliberate reflection but can be mined to reveal your intrinsic, perhaps hidden, dharmic desires. Your history of regrets and yearnings has been recorded in your memory bank. We are born with the power of recall. In Ayurveda this power is named *tarpaka kapha*—the internal record keeper or memory retriever. When we process our emotions regularly through reflection, they are fuel that gets digested and burned into light, generating empowering memories. The light is insight for the vision of who you might become next. As you process your yearnings and regrets, you actually rewrite your memories, updating your records by creating new neural pathways.

When you don't process your emotions, especially difficult emotions such as regret and fear, the mental records become ruts that slow your evolution, reinforcing neural pathways that lead to who you've already been. Updated records hasten your progress and ease your path forward.

As a human being, you were born with the most sacred technology in the known universe: emotions. Your emotions are an essential part of your intelligence, and they overlay your yearnings and regrets, which can guide you to transform your current experiences into your next chapter. If you own your distant and immediate past, you become more integrated—and in that integrity, you are able to design an even brighter future.

Unearthing your dreams starts with articulating your yearnings. Yearning is the voice of your becoming, leading you to do the hard work. Although it might seem paradoxical, by examining your yearnings and regrets, you unlock access to your next level of conscious becoming.

Empower Your Yearning

Over the next week, keep a yearning journal. Even if you aren't a "journaler," commit to this practice. Set a timer—two minutes will get you started. (Also, use your notebook or notetaking app throughout your day to capture insights.)

Record your desires and longings. Note your irritations and your frustrations. As you write, allow your stream-of-consciousness thoughts to take over. Ramble. In the rambling, you are unraveling. The threads you unravel will knit themselves into insights, into a vision of the way forward.

In your unraveling, you are unearthing buried dreams. Your rational mind is of little use here. For most of us, our rational minds are overdeveloped and get in the way. Your mind might even drown out the voice of your heart or your body. Be curious. Dig deep. You are unleashing your dharma by excavating unattended desires.

Next, imagine tomorrow as an uncarved block. What would a terrific day feel like? What would happen? What wouldn't happen?

If you are disconnected from your desire, if years of suppression have left you numb, don't sweat it. You might have been trained to fear your desire. Fear causes constriction, which blocks flow. To transmute your fear into curiosity, start with the small stuff. What do you want to eat tomorrow? What clothes in your closet are your current favorites? What lit you up today? Who brightens your day? What do you want to experience tomorrow?

As you do this practice daily for the next few weeks or months, notice how small desires start to expose your bigger dharma. You can also use the questions at the end of this chapter to jump-start your yearning journal. ■

THE EVOLUTIONARY EFFICIENCY OF ALCHEMIZING REGRET

Have you ever met someone who says they have no regrets? Did you believe them? Does that perspective serve their evolution or encourage a level of complacency? I've found that when we deny or bury our regrets, we short-shrift digesting a regret into a lesson learned.

Your regrets hold wisdom. Befriend your regrets. When you mine your regrets, you refine ore into shiny gold insights that light your path. If you're blocked from your next purpose, your next identity evolution, you'll definitely want to mine your regrets.

You "digest" your regrets through reflection, which unearths the deep longing to fulfill your core needs of connection, intimacy, and personal evolution. This spurs self-compassion. When you mine your regrets, you can assimilate your prior ignorance in order to grow your wisdom. Digested regrets shine the light on smarter actions based on what you know now. By mining regrets, you get to see the common traps you might inadvertently, yet repetitively, set for yourself. You become less likely to regret the next chapter of your future as you hone your intuition, which might have sensed previous traps a mile away.

At the end of the day, after I turn out the light, I replay my day. As I'm celebrating the "good things" that happened, I also mine for regrets. When I replay a regret, even a small one, such as, "I wish I hadn't said that," I rewrite the memory with what would have been a better response, such as, "I could have said this." This small rewrite in my memory generates a better neural pathway that paves the way for a smarter future—a more integrated gut, mind, and heart. It dissolves regressed patterns such as emotional eating or drinking or smoking. This new pathway keeps me from dwelling on past regressions because I'm putting my hands on the steering wheel of tomorrow by digesting and learning from today. Taking a few moments at the end of the day to digest regret rewires the thinking patterns. For me, often the insights give way to actions I need to take the next day to live a more aligned life. Plus, the benefits of better neural pathways with this short end-of-day practice increase with time.

Neuroplasticity is the ability of your brain to change throughout your life. A *Psychology Today* article explains the connection between neuroplasticity and personal evolution: "It may be possible to carve out a fresh and unworn path for your thoughts to travel upon. One could speculate that this process opens up the possibility to reinvent yourself and move away from the status quo."[5] It's possible to update your brain and nervous system to work smarter by being more informed about who you are becoming.

In the next exercise, you'll digest your past to generate power and direction for your future. The power comes from transforming regret into lessons learned. You'll write your yearning and regret history to discover your patterns and your common traps. Through assimilating yearnings and regrets, you'll uncover essential weaknesses you can transform by turning them into strengths. In the end, you'll have more insight into the direction you're heading. You will have alchemized your view of your past and rewired your memories so that your past becomes even more progressive and positive for your future. The point isn't to dwell on regret but rather to transform emotion-laden regrets into intelligent fuel for the fire of your growth. Marshall Goldsmith points out in his book *Triggers: Becoming the Person You Want to Be* that if we embrace regret, including the pain that comes with facing how we've failed ourselves or hurt the people we love with our past choices, it becomes "one of the most powerful feelings guiding us to change." Goldsmith reminds us that no one is exempt from this humbling emotion.[6] Within regret is a sacred opportunity to catalyze buried emotion into dynamic learning.

Digest Your Yearning and Regret History

Set your timer for thirty minutes. Sketch your history visually using stick figures, words, or icons. Start with your earliest childhood memories of regret. When did you first experience regret as a child or young adult? What choices led to this emotion? Assess what your circumstances were, and consider how you got there. Notice: Do you have compassion for yourself at that age? How does it feel to recognize, or re-cognize, your regret?

What were your deepest longings as a teenager? How did you fail yourself or someone else? What did you long for in relationships? What did you envision for your future? What was important to you that you didn't honor with your actions? Were there any buried treasures in there that later resurfaced? What regrets do you have from your teen years?

As you go through this exercise, you might feel your brain rewiring your history; you might notice an improved version or neural pathway of memory. Perhaps forgotten dreams are resurfacing. In reintegrating your history, you are becoming more whole, interconnected. You are maturing your cellular integrity and updating neural pathways, memory by memory, by processing your yearnings and regrets.

Keep going. What happened to you as a young adult? What were your great disappointments? Under disappointment, you can discover a gold mine of yearning. What did your family, friends, or coworkers not see in you? What did you hide? What do you regret about your own behaviors or decisions during that time?

Now, notice how owning your regret points the way to core personal lessons learned and triggers your desire to do better.

Take a moment to honor what regret can teach you when you pause to notice its intelligence to steer your future. Regret hones your intuition. Generate waves of compassion for yourself as a learning, caring, and ever-evolving human being.

Transformation—or your personal evolution—is accelerated by self-compassion. In this process, recognize your efforts to learn, to evolve, and to shape-shift by owning your experiences and absorbing your lessons learned. In this way, you are recovering the reflection-and-closure part of the natural cycle, where the gems of your future are hidden. Be bold and gentle in owning the good, the bad, and the ugly in your history.

Simultaneously you are expanding your capacity for self-compassion as well as empathy and connectivity in your core relationships. When you become more whole, you empower those in your life to become more whole.

Keep going.

What are your regrets from your mature adult experiences? What are your yearnings? See the cycles. Notice the yearnings without shame or judgment.

You'll notice as you move through this book that more memories will surface. Memories will manifest regrets and underlying yearnings. If you stop to add them to your sketch, you will digest them. You are updating your records, rewriting your hard drive, mobilizing your power of tarpaka kapha. In the process, you will more completely and accurately know yourself and the nature of your next purpose. ∎

YOUR SKEPTIC AND YOUR DEEPER DREAM

In addition to the voices of yearning and regret, as part of your human operating system, you are also blessed with the voice of the skeptic. The job of the skeptical voice in your head is to question and doubt. Your skeptic can be employed to make your next purpose and identity real by helping you invest your attention, time, and money wisely. In this section, you'll learn how to channel your skeptic for critical thinking to support you in making the difficult decisions along the way, which will be especially necessary later as you master fire element (vision-planning) and air element (time).

Yet, beware: if your skeptic gets too much airtime, you won't follow your heart. Your tender dreams reside in your heart. When it comes to disrupting your attempts to take action, the skeptic is renowned for putting the cart before the horse. The cart before the horse conversation—putting *how* before *what exactly*—is the skeptic's bad habit. When allied with self-doubt, the skeptic can ensure that no tender dream gets sufficient protection and attention to be elevated into vision-planning. The skeptic can leverage logic and reasons to squash dreams. If you dream big enough, deep enough, or challenging enough, your inner skeptic comes up with handfuls of factual evidence for why you could never nourish the dream to fruition.

The nature of deep, unearthed dreams is that they are not yet real. The person you will be when your next purpose becomes reality is not the person you are today. In the process of aligning your actions with your dreams, your character must evolve, shape-shift, and ascend to next-level integrity. Notably, the logic of your inner skeptic is based on your past, not your future.

To get to know your skeptic, *pause. Ask yourself: What cart are you putting before which horse?* Do you want to close or open a relationship, a venture, a career, a personal pattern? Are you skeptical of how it might all play out? Do you want to try a new way of earning money but are risk averse? Do you want to be an asset to your community but already don't have enough time in the day?

What does your skeptic keep you from doing? To trigger your skeptic, try truing your dreams or thinking of a bigger, brighter future because "playing small" won't trigger your skeptic. What is beyond your wildest dreams? That is sure to trigger your skeptic. If you can hear your skeptical voice, you can deal with it *before* it sabotages your action plan by unconsciously distracting you. Getting to know your skeptic now will save you time and frustration later.

Pause. Ask yourself: What dream is big enough to trigger my skeptic? What reoccurring thoughts or emotions does my skeptic use to disrupt my dreams?

Answering this question and living from that truth is the path of living your life, and bringing your potential, awake.

As you connect with the voices of your yearning, your regret, and your skeptic, you become more whole. During the course of this book, you will befriend your yearning, your regret, and your skeptic. These parts of your humanity are predictors, diviners, and forecasters of the Mastery of You program results. Flip these voices upside down and inside out to shine the light on your dharma.

WILLINGNESS VERSUS READINESS AND WHAT HAPPENS WHEN YOU REFUSE THE QUEST

The danger of not befriending your yearning, regret, and skeptic is that you don't heed the call of dharma, or your ambition. As a result, you could trap yourself in an increasingly restrictive and degenerative negative feedback loop. Not wanting to do what's on your schedule; a repetitive feeling of anxiety, depression, or frustration; or a feeling that your core relationships and career are stuck is a sign of the trap.

Joseph Campbell, a comparative mythology scholar and author whose reverberating advice was to "follow your bliss," describes what happens when one refuses the call to life's adventure: "Refusal of the summons converts the adventure into its negative. Walled in boredom, hard work, or 'culture,' the subject loses the power of significant affirmative action and becomes a victim to be saved. His flowering world becomes a wasteland of dry stones and his life feels meaningless. . . . All he can do is create new problems for himself and await the gradual approach of his disintegration."[7] Clearly, a refusal to attend to your next purpose and emergent identity is high stakes—it could have a pretty dark outcome. Complacency, or seeking the comfortable and the familiar, becomes a jail. Courage shrinks in the face of risk, of the unknown.

However, if you missed the boat on your dharma, there is another right behind it. You can always trade the trap of the comfortable or familiar for the unknown of the quest. In doing so, you expand your horizons. Opportunity is always knocking on your door along the path to self-mastery. Yet, readiness *isn't* an indicator of the right time to heed the call of initiation into your next chapter. There is no such thing as ready because readiness requires a comfort that is never present in meeting the demands of the quest. Paradoxically, readiness is earned through the process of who you will become via the adventure. Only at the end—the hero's return—will you be ready for the quest you just fulfilled. Mythic scholars are clear that those who become great, who heed the call to the quest, display *willingness*, not readiness, for a brighter future. So, if you don't feel ready, you're not alone. Take your own willingness and unreadiness as a predictor that you're in the right place at the right time.

THE COMPLEXITY OF A LIFE OF MEANING IN THE MODERN AGE

If it were only one quest, you might be thinking. Your dreams might be complex and multidimensional. For example, you might be "on purpose" in your family life, your self-care, and your relationships, yet your community impact and life's work might feel hollow. Often some parts of life are on track, and other parts are off the rails.

I learned from Barbara Marx Hubbard, grandmother of *Evolutionaries*, that although we can plant and water the seeds of ideas, we can't know when they'll take root, sprout, grow in spurts, flower, fruit, or abundantly reseed. We have a lifetime to live into various dharmas, or purposes. You intuitively sense your most desirable ideas and dreams, but you can't always estimate the time frame for implementation.

Often when life changes fast, your purpose pivots. One part dies as another breaks through the shell. A breakdown shatters the old identity, begetting a breakthrough. And then, of course, there are the times of latency, of waiting for clarity, of just putting one foot in front of the other.

You might be in a "family phase" of purpose, in which relationships, self-care, and family take center stage. During this phase, you might be frustrated about missing out on your "life's work." Yet, if you have too many irons in the fire, none of them get hot enough to bend. The Master of You program and the exercises in this book will lead you to focus on the best use of your time and energy while you are building your resilience and adaptability. Rest assured that as you follow this system, the seeds you most want to bear fruit will do so at the right time.

THE PARADOX OF EVOLVING AND BEING

Life naturally orients you toward growth—toward a bigger, brighter, and better future. This requires continual personal transformation. Yet, herein lies a paradox: the highly conscious people feel the pull to become greater versions of themselves while simultaneously feeling that they are already enough, complete, whole, healed, and fulfilled. Some call this awareness of tranquil wholeness "the ground of being." Others describe it as the experience of *beingness*. This experience of beingness is always available if we remember to be aware of it. Wisdom traditions guide us into beingness with practices such as sitting or walking in silence, prayer, breathing, singing, and chanting.

The yogis use a number of terms to describe the always available experience of the ground of being: *purna*, or the fullness of being; *svatantrya*, or the freedom and the unlimited expansiveness of being; and *shivaya*, or the auspicious, the favorable—indicating that the experience of beingness is inherently subtly positive, not neutral. By taking a moment to go inward, a person can access the experience of ease, inner fullness, and a sense of all-rightness. A deep freedom of being infused with the positivity inherent in the force and intelligence of life becomes tangible. Personal evolution, or dharma—the work of becoming—is balanced by pausing to root your awareness in beingness. Exercises in many chapters of this book awaken your breath to anchor your journey of becoming by tapping into beingness. Take a moment to remember that you are free both to be and to become. Notice how one pulls your awareness inward and the other outward.

If we orient ourselves only from a place of not-enoughness, or desiring more, we exhaust ourselves and eclipse the joy of the ride. You are intrinsically enough as you are. More time, more money, more intimacy, more credibility, more success without the knowledge that it's all okay, it's all already enough, or it's all good right now create dissatisfaction, greed, and isolation. In *Master of You*, you orient yourself from the perspective that you are already whole and complete and enough *and* that you are evolving. Pause for a moment to ponder the paradox: the serenity of being and the adventure of becoming.

The yogis call the game of becoming a better you *lila*. *Lila* describes the spirit of the game of life, the natural delight in creation, including your next self-invention. Notice for a moment how you feel when you take your self-mastery path playfully, knowing there will be interesting characters and situations that arise along your path. What if you can take all this a little less seriously, with a little more delight? What if in the lessons you'll learn along the way, you can see the playfulness of the divine, or a playful quality in the evolutionary force itself? Would that serve you? We'll return to this concept, especially when the journey becomes arduous!

Through the reflection you've started in this chapter, you are shifting from existing pattern to potential. *Master of You* helps you learn to slow down the points of time between your choices. In yoga language, behavioral or mental ruts are called *samskaras*, or grooves made from repetitive mental and emotional habits. Your thinking ruts are naturally habitual, perpetuated by the whirlwind of busy days and aggravated by not enough pausing to reflect and realign the course of your next action. Out of the rut, your perspective changes. I hope this chapter boosts you out of the habitual thinking ruts and into liminal thinking. Building new neural pathways allows you to feel the buzz of potentiality.

A life that matters greatly is a process. The more you trust your process and cheer yourself on, the more you access the grace of your own becoming. As you become aware of your deeper dreams, you can sense the new skills these dreams will require. As you endeavor to acquire these skills, you become a better version of your self, more capable than ever. Your identity evolves. Notably, you simultaneously become a boon to others on their paths of becoming.

Welcome to the game of your life, where you get to be you, dream bigger, and grow (see Figure 1.3).

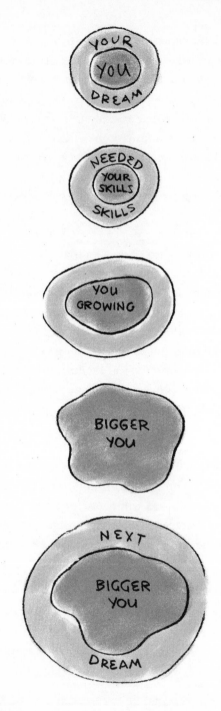

Figure 1.3 Bigger you

YOUR TO-DO LIST

○ Journal before bed about your even more desirable dreams.

○ Pay homage to your voice of yearning.

○ Digest your regrets at the end of the day.

○ Trigger your skeptic so you can observe what habitually keeps you from acting on your deeper dreams.

○ Witness yourself through a lens of compassion.

○ Reflect on the following questions:

  • What would you do with an uncarved block of time to do whatever you want? How long of an uncarved block of time do you want?

  • As you go through the day, ask yourself: Is there anything I'd rather be doing or not doing?

  • What does your ideal home look like? Feel like? Where is it located?

  • What do you wish were different in your life?

  • What are you attracted to? Which foods? Which people? Which ideas?

  • Where or when in life have you numbed your yearning? Which yearnings do you allow, and which do you repress?

  • What recurring thoughts, or sentences, does your skeptic use to disrupt your dreams?

- Can you awaken your willingness for the journey ahead?

- Can you drop into the experience of beingness?

- What dream are you unearthing now?

2

INNOVATING WITH THE FIVE PRIMORDIAL ELEMENTS

Have you ever sacrificed one part of yourself to develop another? A common example is focusing less on improving body habits as you pursue your career or raise your family. Another is putting your spiritual development on the back burner to put food on the table. In the Master of You program, no part is left behind. In order to holistically create the daily experience you want next, you must awaken the power of all five of the elements. In leaving no element behind, you can develop all parts of yourself, including building resilience in your body, awakening your intuition, following your spirit, and fulfilling even greater worldly ambitions.

To awaken the power of the elements, you need to access your intuitive, symbolic, and even spiritual awareness. Our modern culture is especially developed in linear, rational thinking. This type of thinking isn't as effective when it comes to accessing the innate intelligence of the five primordial elements as experiential concepts. Keep this in mind throughout the book—we are orienting ourselves conceptually rather than scientifically. Therefore, we'll go on a journey in this chapter to stir your awareness, your intuition, and your everyday experience of the five elements in hopes of preparing you for a much deeper dive, element by element, in part 2. To awaken your awareness of the powers of the elements, we start with their origin—the life-force energy, from which the universe was born.

In yoga, the origin of the elements is explained as the universal energy becoming matter. This universal energy, shakti, is infused with the intelligence of the life force. The universal intelligence activated that force to become matter; simplicity became complexity and uniformity became diversity as the energy manifested itself into the five elements. The five elements became the basic building blocks of our cosmos and generated the infinite expressions of life forms. Our ancient ancestors from myriad cultures described the life-force energy coming into form through the elements: from space (essence), to air (movement), to fire (transformation), to water (cohesion), to earth (matter). All human ancestral cultures venerated the energy that generated the "big bang" of our universe, the energy still unfolding today. The yogis call the life-force energy *shakti*; the Japanese call it *ki*; the Chinese, *chi*; the Native Americans, *divine spirit* or *medicine*; and the Christians, *Holy Ghost*. The Polynesians call it *mana*; the Jews, *ruach*; and the Muslims, *baraka*.

Our ancestors perceived the elements as the basic ingredients of everything. The elements were essential in the ancient sciences of medicine, philosophy, astronomy, and religion. The life force in the elements isn't just a concept, as it might seem to modern humans. Contemporary culture has lost this understanding of the elements. Modern science and medicine have missed the mark on the profound, holistic, and intuitive wisdom of the elements, dismissing five-element theory as primitive. Yet, reconnecting with the five elements leads to deeper intuition and holistic awareness. The elements around you and within you become tangible, malleable building blocks of reality, revealing how to design the next season of your life, as I'll show you in part 2.

Ayurveda, similar to other indigenous lifeways, is both an ancient and emergent wisdom tradition, focused on a life of radiant longevity.[1] Ayurveda is an ancient noetic science. Noetic science is based on cultivating inner wisdom through direct knowing, coupled with observing and experimenting with the world around us (known as science). Ayurveda identifies the elements as concepts or principles (as opposed to periodic table elements). Ayurvedic physician Vasant Lad, author of eleven books on the subject, explains how the elements are the basis of everything, from the planet itself to human beings: "Man is a microcosm of the universe, and therefore, the five basic elements present in all matter also exist within each individual."[2] Lad goes on to explain this foundational concept: "More than physical elements, the five elements represent ideas that are fundamental to nature and matter. The five elements are collections of qualities that together form the building blocks of nature. If a person truly understands the five elements, the doorway of knowledge opens to understanding creation itself."[3]

In forsaking the intrinsic wisdom of the elements, we modern people have disempowered our bodies, our daily life rhythms, our prosperity, our futures, and our progeny. As a culture we are under-rested and over-fed, from our elders to our youth. One in seven Americans is estimated to have an autoimmune disease; women constitute 75 percent of these, and that number is growing.[4] Around half of American adults are in debt, and that number is also growing.[5] The Master of You program repairs this rift, guiding you experientially. The more fully you understand the elements intuitively, conceptually, and experientially, the more skillfully and naturally you'll use the primordial building blocks to live a life aligned to your purpose, personal integrity, and unique meaning. Unlock the wisdom and power in the elements and you access the knowledge of how to design yourself and your world.

To start, turn your attention to noticing the elements right now. Your feelings are an easy access point to connect with the five elements. As you read about the elements, notice what resonates. For example, do you feel naturally at ease, light in your body, and relaxed in your daily schedule? Then you are accessing the power of space. Space element also generates inclusivity in our relationships. So, on the flip side, if you feel trapped in your life or if you are wired and tired, overfed, and feeling excluded, you aren't protecting your space element, so space can't empower your life. This is because space's chief characteristic is expansion outward from the center; it has no density or heat. Earth, the densest and most material of the elements, gives you the qualities of endurance, resilience, and stability. If you have activated earth's powers, you are sure-footed, levelheaded, and steady. You command the space and opportunities around you. If you haven't activated earth element, you will tend toward being indecisive, anxious, and perhaps fragile. Or, if your earth element is stubborn and stuck, you have anchored yourself in your own limitations by not evolving with the times.

Fire engages friction to transform, generating light for the vision required to transcend obstacles. If you are awake to your purpose and clear in your actions, and if you are able to transform tough circumstances into opportunities for growth, your fire element is strong. If fire element is underdeveloped in you, you will not feel on track with your goals and might grow complacent when a situation demands firm follow-through and overcoming obstacles. Air, which can move in any direction, has the freedom and flexibility of mobility. So, if you are frequently hurrying, late, or behind on your projects, you are out of sync with air element. If you feel like a master of your time, centered yet available and adaptable for what arises, on target yet spontaneous, you have strong command of air element.

Water element requires us to surrender our will, our knowing, and our ways to a higher power. Water requires us to bow our minds to our hearts, our heads to our bellies—to surrender to the process of transformation, however that might go and wherever that might lead. Water will at times forcefully invite you to embody the weightier lessons you have learned. Water will escort you to new levels of your own depth, maybe even to the point where you know the source of who you are. With water's intelligence, you move slowly enough for people to feel your presence and compassion, which creates a sense of acceptance, connection, and even solace. This is because water element brings people together and helps us absorb the harder lessons learned in life, through the qualities of cohesion and flow and the weightiness of gravity. Yet, if you haven't developed water element within, it can suppress the vision of fire element and the adaptability of air element, leaving you anchored and isolated under the weight of their worlds. Equally disempowering, you could drift through your life without engaging the responsibilities that lead to the depth of character and future you want to cultivate.

With only this brief introduction, you already have some literacy regarding the elements. Ultimately, you're aiming for a deeply embodied experience of your five elements, and that is the goal of *Master of You*. You want to unleash the ancient powers of the cosmos, of the life force within the elements and within yourself. The five elements are a framework to unlock ever-increasing levels of self-knowledge, universal wisdom, and the empowerment that comes with both. Your aim is not to "balance" your elements. Your aim is to behold their powers within your spirit, mind, and body.

In the next exercise you'll get reacquainted with the elements, their language, and their powers.

You Are the Elements

If you would like to listen to this exercise, you can access a recording at masterofyou.us/workbook.

Take a few slow, deep breaths to connect with the life force and the consciousness that informs this base of universal energy. Notice how your body and mind feel after a moment of slower, deeper breathing.

To connect with the elements, stand up. With your hands, pat your physical body. That is your earth element. Look outside and notice the land, the trees, the buildings—anything with form. That is also earth element. Notice the structure and solidity.

Next, notice water. Gently squeeze your body with your hands. Notice your liquidity—the squishy nature of your tissue. Exhale on the palm of your hand, and notice the moisture. About 60 percent of your body is water.[6] Look outside, and see if there are clouds in the sky, puddles, streams, rivers, or any other signs of water.

Then, feel your skin around your middle. Notice your warmth. That is fire element. Look in a mirror and notice the light in your eyes. Exhale on the palm of your hand, and notice the heat. That is also fire. Look outside, and notice the daylight or night. Notice the sun or the stars. That is fire element.

Next, notice air. Feel your body inhale and exhale. Feel your pulse. Your cells are bathed in constant motion, even when sleeping. Exhale on the palm of your hand, and notice the breeze. That is air element. Look outside, and notice the wind on the leaves of the tree. That is air.

Finally, look outside as far as your eyes can see. That is the expansive nature of our planet in space. That is space element. Now, close your eyes to look within yourself. Perhaps you can notice a quiet stillness behind all the motion, the heat, the moisture, and your density. You are accessing space element. ■

YOU ARE THE COSMOS AND THE ELEMENTS

"Cosmos" in the context of *Master of You* refers to the expanding multiverse, including our planet, galaxy, solar system, universe, and the 13+ billion years of the evolution of consciousness into form, which created and continues to evolve us. It includes the blood that courses through our bodies as well as our multiple levels of intelligence, our personal evolution, and our misgivings. The cosmos encapsulates our collective origin, evolution, and next becoming. We cannot be divided from the cosmos, which created us, in the same way we cannot be separated from the history that evolved matter into humans. Noetic sciences see the human being as a *holon*—simultaneously a singular expression of the whole cosmos and a part of it. You can perceive your self as a representation of the whole of the cosmos and as a miniscule particle in it. This cosmos-centric consciousness opens us to thinking big and testing small—a concept we'll see later in the ethos of Master of You (chapter 3).

Every cell is also a holon, and every holon—or microrepresentative of the cosmos—contains all five elements. You have a unique constitution, made up of varying percentages of the elements, as your baseline. You also have a personal purpose and native genius that can be described in terms of the elements. The elements that appear in higher amounts within you make you different and are responsible for your "patterns"—your physical, mental, emotional, and spiritual propensities. To shape yourself, unleash your power and next purpose, and expand your personality, you'll want to learn more about your constitution.

Master Your Constitution: Learn the Doshas

Your unique constitution, including your personality, is dominated by specific characteristics of the underlying elements. For instance, if you tend to have a lighter, more enthusiastic personality and be small boned and thin-skinned, those characteristics are shaped by the elements of air and space.

We can use parts of speech—nouns, adjectives, and verbs—to understand how Ayurveda explains the elements. You can think of the elements as nouns—they are static principles. The qualities of the elements—their characteristics—are adjectives (such as light, heavy, warm, damp, etc.). When the elements become activated, they turn into forces, or actions. These are like verbs. The catabolic force of movement happens when air activates space; this is *vata*. Fire and water become the metabolic force of transformation; this is *pitta*. Water activates earth as the anabolic force that nourishes life; this is *kapha*. These synergies enliven us and influence our physical, mental, and emotional tendencies. Derived from the elements and referred to as *doshas*, these synergies, or forces—vata, pitta, and kapha—are at play in your body and mind, your schedule, and even the atmosphere of a room. For example, you might hear someone say that they are pitta dosha (which could mean they tend to have a fiery personality and oily skin) or that the energy of a place feels very vata (which could mean it feels cold, dry, and disorganized). If someone said their schedule was kapha-like, it could mean it is full and dull and feels heavy.

As you recognize how the forces in this triad come alive in your personality and purpose, you can awaken your dharma and leadership style. An Ayurvedic personality test (see Yogahealer.com/quiz) can guide you to identify your constitution (your primary dosha or doshas). Table 2.1 is also a good place to start. Table 2.1 is a decoder you can use to identify your dominant elements, qualities, forces, personality, purpose, and body type. Mark it as a reference for discovering your elemental pattern.

→

Element or Building Block of Life Force (Nouns)	Qualities of Life (Adjectives)	Triadic Forces (Verbs)	Dosha (Sanskrit for Force)	Personality	Leadership Inclination	Body Type (when at optimal weight)
space air	subtle, cold, expanding, light, ethe-ric, mobile, clear, dry, rough, cold, light	force that moves and communicates: catabolic	vata	curious, enthusiastic, energizing, alert, quick to learn, flexible, forgiving, sensitive, talkative, unconventionally expressive or creative	inspirational, unconventional, and creative leader	light, long, thin or narrow frames, lithe, may naturally look interesting or eccentric, long face, small or tall, cold body temperature, thin dry skin, tends toward sensitivity
fire water	hot, sharp, light, liquid, spreading, oily, wet, smooth, slow, cool, sticky, cloudy	force that digests and transforms: metabolic	pitta	focused, direct, analytical, intense, powerful intellect, inspiring, precise, strategic, visionary	visionary and strategic leader	medium height, weight, muscle tone, angular face, strong digestion and appetite, warm body temperature, tends toward inflammation
earth	heavy, dull, dense, stable, gross	force that builds structure, cohesion and lubricates: anabolic	kapha	relaxed, trusting, loyal, comfortable, patient, understanding, accepting, supportive	managerial and operational leader	strong build, denser body mass, round face and eyes, thick hair, cool moist skin, sleeps soundly, tends toward lethargy

To understand the elements, familiarize yourself with their consistent qualities. Earth is heavy, tangible, stable, unmoving, and cool. Water is wet, heavy, smooth, cool, cloudy, and flowing. Fire is hot, sharp, subtle, oily, and light. Air is mobile, dry, inconsistent, light, clear, cold, rough, and subtle. Space is the most subtle and expansive—the lightest, clearest, and coldest. The elements are categorized along various spectra of density, friction (or temperature), moisture, and mobility, to name a few. These spectra run the range of opposite qualities, such as light to heavy, dry to wet, cold to hot, clear to cloudy, subtle to gross, rough to smooth, sharp to dull, mobile to stagnant. The qualities help you identify where you are and if you need to correct your course. For example, if you are traveling, you might notice that your skin dries out, you might feel anxiety about making your next flight, or you might forget your phone in a bathroom. Dry, mobile, and inconsistent are attributes related to the movement of travel, dominated by air and space elements.

USING THE FIVE-ELEMENT SYSTEM TO MASTER YOUR HOME, BODY, AMBITION, TIME, AND FLOW

In my career of passing forward the wisdom of Ayurveda and yoga through innovative courses, I came to see that the five-element system was hidden in plain view. I internalized this system to design my household, my body, my time, and my career. I then built an online course around it and tested the system with the members.

A good curriculum is a system that accesses a specific dimension of learning. It is also a model that fosters growth toward higher, more integrated levels by having learners practice certain competencies, often in a *krama*, or order, that enables efficiency and ease. Only those with the new skills and capacities access the next level, or dimension. This is true for all endeavors, from sports to mathematics, at which one improves in stages. A good model codifies order out of complexity, making it navigable for others to use for advancement. Those who thoroughly engage with the Master of You system get the best results the fastest—meaning goals they'd struggled for years to achieve become reachable. More important than their reaching individual goals, they can apply the system to continually improve who they become next. "Once a good model gets inside you, it can inform and guide you throughout a lifetime," say Bob Anderson and William Adams in *Mastering Leadership*.[7] Soon, what you thought was beyond your capacity becomes a matter of applying the system. As behavior researcher James Clear points out in *Atomic Habits*, "You do not rise to the level of your goals. You fall to the level of your systems."[8]

The Master of You system starts with space, the subtlest element, because it is the easiest to influence. You will gain quick traction with your deeper dreams by shaping your space and enhancing your living environments to align with who you want to become next. The opposite of space is earth, which we focus on second.

In working with earth, you will shape your physical body rhythms with the daily habits that support deep rejuvenation and peak performance. From earth, we'll go to fire. By that point in this system, you will be inspired, alight with your next ambitions, and eager to set your vision. In working with the mental intensity of fire element, from your vision you develop a strategy to form your best plan.

With your plan, you will move into the field of time, the air element. You'll upgrade your calendar to align to your plan. Naturally, challenges and issues will surface, indicating that you have landed in the depth of water element.

In water element, additional competencies and higher levels of personal integration not visible when you built your strategy will be required. By revealing and befriending these issues and developing the competencies necessary, these shadows become the light that powers your next wave of growth. Master of You is an iterative system. Certain elements in which you already have competencies will be easy for you, and others will escort you into uncharted territory and untapped capacities. In the next section, you will uncover your *current* status with the five elements.

SPACE, EARTH, FIRE, AIR, WATER

Let's go through the five-element assessment. As you read the lists of competencies for mastering each element, note which ones you most want to master right now, which are current strengths, and which are blind spots.

Space

A master of space element experiences unencumbered personal freedom and creativity. To get there, you will shape the spaces you inhabit with intentional design. Space is the surrounding area—the vibrational atmosphere between structures. The subtlest element in the system, space is referred to as ether because it has an etheric quality. What is in a space alters the atmosphere. You want the right amount of space and the right quality of space. For example, when you overeat, you decrease space in your stomach, disrupting good digestion. When you overcrowd your desk or your calendar, you decrease focus. Your living spaces, your working spaces, and even how you organize your refrigerator or the trunk of your car reflect your relationship with space element. Notice the atmosphere when you walk into a room. The environments we create are determined by how we organize and fill the space. This is at the forefront of behavioral science, explains author and executive leadership coach Marshall Goldsmith: "If we do not create and control our environment, our environment creates and controls us."[9] How the space is constructed facilitates certain behaviors. If your fridge is clean and organized with ready-to-eat vegetables and fruit in plain view and prepared foods at the back, you will be more likely to eat fresh vegetables and fruits. If you leave your desk with a short, prioritized to-do list, you are likely to take aligned action when you return.

As you read the space competencies below, what do you desire to experience next?

MASTER OF SPACE (HOME)

○ You design your spaces intentionally to improve
  your mental clarity, focus, and intuition.

○ You shape your space to guide and support the habits
  you want next, making habit evolution a breeze.

○ You seasonally organize and refresh your spaces.

○ Your spaces reflect your values and your personal ethos.

○ You have no clutter, resulting in an energetic
  efficiency from desire to action.

○ All of your possessions add value, meaning,
  and direction to your life.

○ When in your spaces, you feel ease, rejuvenation,
  creativity, and expansiveness.

Earth

The most physical element in the system is earth. Earth is all
about how you live in sync with your body's needs—your body
rhythms—and intentionally design your body through your habits.
Just as the planet is the foundation of our shared existence, your body
is the foundation of your existence. Your past habits and experiences
have generated the body you have today. In mastering earth element,
you honor your body rhythms and grow your immune strength. You
reinforce and continually improve the best habits for your body to
steer toward radiant longevity. Like Mother Nature, earth element is
characterized by cycles that beget resilience. Which earth competencies do you want?

MASTER OF EARTH (BODY)

○ You befriend and strengthen your body with
rhythmic eating, moving, and sleeping.

○ Your bones are carrying the right amount of muscle
and fat for you at this stage of your life.

○ You have strong digestion that contributes to stable energy,
a focused mind, positive emotions, and deep sleep.

○ You expand your daily repertoire of functional movement.

○ You take movement breaks a few times a day
rather than or in addition to "working out."

○ You consistently improve and refine your habits to optimize
your future body and power your next purpose.

Fire

From intentionally working with space and earth, your self-directedness, confidence, and informed optimism expand. Insights and potentialities arise as you surround yourself with highly functional spaces and strengthen your body rhythms. Fire generates heat and light. With light you can see, envision possibilities, and visualize a brighter future. The focused mental fire discerns which actions lead to outcomes and which causes generate the desired effects. This discernment of all possibilities for a clarified, specified vision requires the burning laser focus of fire element. With fire, you develop your best strategy and then your best possible plan. Which fire competencies resonate with you?

MASTER OF FIRE (AMBITION)

◯ You author your life.

◯ You align your life goals for deeper purpose and meaning, repeatedly expanding beyond who you have already been.

◯ You invest your time up front in vision, strategy, and planning to meet your goals.

◯ You investigate the critical issues standing between you and your goals.

◯ You build strategy based on your critical issues.

◯ You reverse-engineer a plan with milestones, aligned actions, and habits that lead to your vision.

◯ You are able to radically develop capacities, skills, and relationships and evolve your identity in line with your goals.

Air

In order to activate vision, movement is required. Movement is the primary quality of air element, and movement measures time. In mastering air element, you increase your competency with the goals you can move forward in a block of time. You'll master structuring your time with distinct choices. Aligning to dharma requires skill development, which you'll need to schedule. Curiosity, the emotional quality of air element, will help you reinvent your calendar in unexpected ways. Wonder gives rise to the experience of bending time—a deeply altered perception of time in which you save time in unexpected ways, opening more freedom in the next chapter of your life. Air element invites you to become the master of your time by scheduling your daily rhythm for peak performance and creativity, fueled by deep rejuvenation and rest. Check off which competencies from air element you want next.

MASTER OF AIR (TIME)

○ You align your body rhythms with the projects that lead to your goals on the calendar.

○ You don't wait until you feel ready; you do the activities you scheduled on your calendar.

○ You avoid distraction and multitasking.

○ You master the daily rhythm of deep rejuvenation and peak performance by blocking your calendar into free time, focus time, and buffer blocks.

○ You create strategic relationships, such as receiving coaching, exchanging mentoring, and delegating tasks to move your goals forward.

○ You schedule time for annual, quarterly, monthly, weekly, and daily planning to tune in to your vision and align your actions.

○ You have alignment meetings with yourself, your family, and your coworkers to structure the week ahead.

Water

Water is the healing element, and it joins your past with your potential. Water heals the rifts, or integrity gaps, and provides cohesion to propel the vision of your future. Unlike fire, which hastens time, water slows time and can be disorienting in its healing process. From its weightiness, cloudiness, and permeability, water escorts you to the depths of your own underworld, like the goddesses Demeter and Persephone in the ancient myths. Water invites us to become smarter over time, bringing to the surface our past naivete and outdated habits and patterns. Just as fire calls us to mental maturity, water calls us to emotional, intuitional, and spiritual maturation and integrated alignment of our spirit, intuition, emotions, thoughts, energy, and body. Water might circulate around us as we integrate our past identities with our emerging identities, updating what we are aware of as well as what we value most. Water's power plumbs uncharted depths in our character. In escorting us to new depths, water helps us heal and resurface as a more integrated human being. Water's end results are ease, flow, and prosperity. Which water competencies do you want?

MASTER OF WATER (INTEGRITY AND FLOW)

○ You follow your desire, even when it leads
through difficult terrain, seeking to understand
the challenges of your next dharma.

○ You are willing to become who it takes—to
expand your capacities and integrity.

○ You understand that your next level of personal
growth is rooted in your next depth of character.

○ You determine the high-impact, low-effort activities that pave
an efficient path to the work that needs to be done next.

○ You generate opportunities to add more value or exchange
more value in your life, which generates financial fluency.

○ When challenges arise, you nourish yourself
with healing breath-body practices.

To become masterful with the elements, you will cycle around and around, season by season, developing greater capacities and becoming the person you've always wanted to be. As Dan Sullivan of Strategic Coach advises, "The moment you have arrived is the perfect time to start out again."[10] You will discover that certain elements are your strong suits, and others are your black holes. With iterations of this process, you become more integrated, which creates another path of potential for the next chapter of your life. This happens continually, with each growth cycle revealing the next challenges. At some point, you will experience this system within you, your thinking, and your actions.

Master of You guides you to invest your attention in yourself and your next purpose. With *Master of You*, you steer your own ship. Ayurveda and yoga—the primary influences of the program—have always been a lighthouse for truth-seekers and those desiring the ultimate human experience. The exercises in the coming chapters will help you integrate the elements and make them come alive in your day-to-day life, their primordial powers underpinning your next ambitions.

Let's do this.

MASTER OF YOU ETHOS

good exercise

B y activating a code of ethics, you can more easily develop habits that reinforce your own values and skillfully navigate tough situations that arise on this journey. The twelve values of the Master of You ethos, outlined in this chapter, arose over time through my leading the online courses, and I noticed that the members who practice them see results faster. You also might find that experimenting with these values influences better choices.

This value system is an ethos—both a skill set and a mindset—and I'll refer to it throughout this book to consciously reinforce the Master of You culture, which facilitates synchronizing your home, your body, and your time with your ambition. Ideally, the Master of You ethos resonates with your personal ethos—the spirit of your way of life, which codifies what you feel is dear, true, and worthy of upholding.

Culture can influence our habits even more than our personal ethos does. Our habits often don't reflect our values. We might value sleep yet cut corners when it comes to bedtime. We might value home-made food yet stock the freezer with prepared foods. Small, innocuous actions, when done repetitively—such as taking your cell phone to bed for an alarm clock—quickly become habits. You might have a value around tech-free time but find that you have a hard time living in alignment with that value. When your actions are in line with your values, or ethos, you have a better shot at attuning your life to a higher purpose. For example, you might highly value quiet time, deep rest, good food, and your best friends, yet you find that your days are too busy to find quiet, you're too wired to sleep deeply, you're eating prepared foods, and you haven't had enough time for friendship. Your values haven't changed, but your actions have. When you do this repeatedly, you form habits that are out of integrity with your values. Being out of integrity with your personal ethos feels bad and off track. This chapter is an experiential tour through the twelve values of the Master of You system, which serve as accelerators on this path of self-mastery. The exercises are super helpful, but if you're in the mood for reading rather than doing, you can always come back to them later.

The cultures we are part of, including global culture, influence our thoughts and our actions, sometimes even more than our values do. Our global political culture can be described as volatile, uncertain, complex, and ambiguous (VUCA). A term commonly used in the business world today by strategists and leadership experts, VUCA was first used by students in the US Army War College in the late 1980s to describe the aftermath of the Cold War.[1] Living in a VUCA world, it's easy to make small, daily choices that are out of alignment with your values. Even eating too much, drinking too much, doing too much, staying up too late, working at a job where you are unhappy, staying in an unhealthy relationship, or taking in too much screen time can tip your balance from resilient to weak. The more clear you are on your own ethos, the smarter you can be in navigating the small choices in daily life influenced by a VUCA culture, which will naturally lead you to become more resilient, more skillful, and more adaptable.

If it resonates with you, print the following ethos list (also available at masterofyou.us/workbook) and put it on your fridge.

THE MASTER OF YOU ETHOS

1. Orient yourself to thrive.

2. Adopt a cosmocentric view.

3. Evolve your identity.

4. Nurture and nourish your five bodies.

5. Heed the rhythm and the cycles.

6. Think big, test small, fail fast, learn always.

7. Invest in you.

8. Embrace a solid B–.

9. Trust your desire.

10. Leverage your strengths.

11. Learn. Mentor. Master. Cocreate.

12. Shift from consumer to collaborator.

As you investigate the twelve values in detail, notice which you can immediately apply to your life.

1. Orient Yourself to Thrive

Orienting yourself to thrive is like having an inner GPS to navigate the small decisions in your day. From what to eat and what to do next to who to have on your phone favorites list, little decisions shape your life and your future direction. When you ask this simple question first: "What orients me to thrive?" you make smarter decisions faster.

For example, imagine you're choosing between going to bed early and watching the next series on Netflix. Which points like a compass toward a better tomorrow? When tougher situations arise, and you feel like a victim of circumstance, ask yourself, "In this situation, how can I orient myself to thrive?" This ethos puts you in the driver's seat.

Orient Yourself to Thrive

Consider your morning routine—from the moment you open your eyes until you go to work or begin projects. Identify one or two small actions you can start tomorrow to orient yourself to thrive, such as sitting in silence for a few minutes, drinking a glass of water as soon as you rise, exercising for fifteen minutes, giving someone a hug, or drinking green juice. Design tomorrow's morning routine to orient your day to thrive. Then, do it. ∎

2. Adopt a Cosmocentric View

Cosmos is the word that consciousness communities use to describe the whole of creation. With a cosmocentric perspective, you sense the universe that created you—universal organization, evolution, and being-ness. Such a perspective zooms out to tap into the organized intelligence and the deep time of a universe expanding for 13.7 billion years. This feeling absorbs the VUCA: rather than volatile, it feels peaceful; rather than uncertain, it feels phenomenal; rather than complex, it feels intelligently ordered; rather than ambiguous, it feels miraculous. Instilling a cosmocentric viewpoint at the very start of your day sets you up with an expanded, inclusive, systems-oriented, proactive, yet peaceful perspective on your daily reality.

We shape our minds by how we direct our attention by choosing perspectives that generate more intelligent ideas and connections. When you zoom out your perspective as far as your brain can experience—into the infinitely expanding universe—paradoxically, you can also better locate your own place in the world, your own center.

The default setting of the oldest part of the human brain, known as the reptilian brain, is myopic. Your instinctive response is to contract the world, resulting in you feeling apart, alone, unsupported, or essentially afraid and desiring the known, certain, safe, and predictable. In a world that has always been unpredictable and scary, it's easy to lose the bigger picture, the curiosity, and the receptivity of the beginner's mind that comes from a perspective in which you are part of an unfathomably larger evolutionary whole.

Yet, the feeling you're after is simultaneously expanded and centered. You can start each day by opening yourself to the experience of infinite possibility, of your true potential, rather than jumping right into your plan for the day.

We can reset our internal operating systems, our nervous systems, to run on the intelligence and universal energy that engineered us—shakti. When we start our days by opening to the great mystery, we get to experience connectivity, insight, and ease. This viewpoint is an iterative skill anyone can develop (and experience immediately) by doing the exercise below.

Adopt a Cosmocentric View

(You can also listen to a recording of this exercise at masterofyou.us/workbook.) After you wake up and before you get out of bed, take a moment to expand your awareness. The morning stillness before the dawn is the time of day when the cosmocentric perspective is most accessible.

First, become aware of deep time. Sense the vastness of the universe that made you. Let your body relax and your attention expand. Become aware of the whole of your life span. Then, expand your awareness to the life spans of your ancestors, and then, to the whole of human history. Then go back to the time of the dinosaurs, to mammals, to multicelled organisms, to single-celled organisms. Next, visualize the evolution of your body; notice the preciousness of your life. Then move your awareness through the history of our planet and creation of the elements: space, air, fire, earth, and water. Then sense into the origin of particles, the origin of space, and then to our cosmos as a whole in its beginning.

Notice the present moment. Relax and expand into your day: allow your awareness to effortlessly organize and order your day ahead, prioritizing, making room for what should be next, giving some space and time to your day. You're proactively prioritizing. Later in the day, if you find yourself in a stress loop, use the stress as an emotional trigger to exhale, inhale, and relax again into the abundance of deep time and space. Then visualize the rest of your day ahead from the cosmocentric perspective. ■

3. Evolve Your Identity

When Odysseus returned from his odyssey after two decades, only his neglected dog recognized him. That is what identity evolution looks like. The heroine's journey is a trip into the next level of you—into your next identity. The call to adventure, the initiation, the pit of despair, the mentor, the triumph, and the return are the heroine's journey. Heeding the call of the journey is making the choice to grow, to change, to make your potential real. The heroine *can't stay the same*, can't get tripped up by the same problems. The heroine's world expands; her personal integrity deepens.

The seasoned heroine knows she is a verb, not a noun, a "becoming," not a personality. She knows that her identity is plastic, evolving. On a fierce growth path, she might hardly recognize herself from two years ago. Her thoughts, ideas, relationships, and consciousness are on a higher plane or another dimension altogether.

The challenges you encounter on your growth path flex and shapeshift your identity. This value is a commitment to expanding, to evolving as you become more capable, more adept at generating the change you want to see in your world.

We can all expect the trials, frustrations, and pitfalls inherent in a heroine's journey. In the next exercise, you will identify (1) who you have been, (2) your call to adventure, and (3) who you are becoming. Your future self is thrilled to have this conversation with you.

Evolve Your Identity: The Superheroine Infographic

Grab some colored pens and two pieces of paper. Drawing skill level required: four-year-old level. You will use one of the pictures you're about to draw throughout the rest of the book (see Figure 3.1). So, if you can't complete this exercise right now, be sure to come back to it—you will need your personal superheroine/superhero infographic throughout the rest of the Master of You process. (You can also download a worksheet for this exercise at masterofyou.us/workbook.)

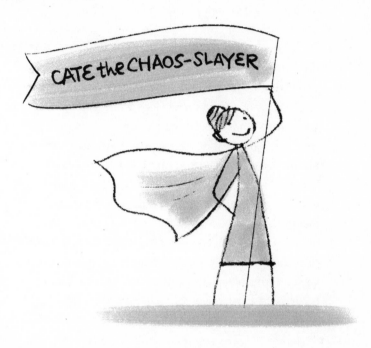

Figure 3.1 Use this dorky image to inspire you to draw yourself as a superheroine or superhero. Give yourself a cape and a name.

1. On the first piece of paper, draw who you are now. What do you look like? What do you feel like? What do you dress like? What skills do you have? What tools do you carry? Who are your friends? What are you reading, studying, and thinking about? What habits do you have automated? What do you eat? Where are your aches and pains? Your frustrations? Your limitations? Include all that comes to mind: use words, arrows, images. Uncover your good, your bad, your ugly.

2. Before drawing the second picture, pause and feel the presence of your call to adventure. Living a life above and beyond your current reality requires something to happen. Feel the call. What are you carving into the block? Remember your deepest dreams. Let them inform your next picture.

3. On your second piece of paper, draw who you will be as the returning victor of your heroine's journey. What does she look like? What does she feel like? What does she dress like? What skills does she have? What tools does she carry? Who are her friends? What is she reading, studying, and thinking about? What habits does she have automated? What does she eat? Add speech bubbles, bullet points, or doodles or create a collage if you are inspired. Make yourself into a superheroine.[2] Give yourself a cape. Give yourself a title or stage name or nickname. In the Vedic (ancient Hindu) tradition, the superheroines (the deities and goddesses) have extra arms. Give yourself as many limbs as necessary to carry all the tools you need.

4. Put your picture on the wall, your bathroom mirror, your fridge, or in your closet—somewhere you will see it every day.

My current superheroine version of me is *Cate, the Legendary Leader*. Embarrassing, right?

My picture has me sporting some funky, Renaissance-era boots with a short flare dress. I have a big pink heart in the center of my chest, and I'm releasing a big pink arrow to hit the target right in front of me. I have a big blue cape that looks regal and blows in the wind. Never mind that I don't have knees and I have an inverted nose—most small children can draw better. What matters is that I have a clear picture of who I'm becoming next.

Your superheroine infographic needs to make sense only to you and represent your best version of your next self. However, I post my picture publicly in my home (and on my course member forum). For achieving goals, making it public is an indispensable strategy. Make yours public so your people can cheer you on, reinforcing the choices and activities that make your hero's journey become reality faster.

You'll use this image as a reference point for identity evolution, so do this exercise before you get to part 2 of this book. You'll return to this exercise with each cycle of the Master of You process. ■

4. Nurture and Nourish Your Five Bodies

The next principle is to care for your whole self. Tendencies turn into automated habits, and in some cases we have automated neglecting things into black holes. As humans, we can develop physical hardiness and also exquisite sensitivity. When we hold these opposite traits simultaneously—through developing ourselves physically, psychically, cognitively, energetically, intuitively, and spiritually—we become more integrated, more adaptable, and more capable. This value helps us maximize our exclusively human technology—the *koshas*, or bodies. Ayurveda describes the five koshas as the layers, or sheaths, of the self. The five bodies are energetic layers, or organizing fields, for how you as a soul get to experience life:

1. Your physical body: Sometimes also called the gross body, this is any tangible part of you that has mass. From blood to bones, nerve, muscle, and skin, this is the body on which you hang your clothes.

2. Your breath body: This is the subtle layer of yourself that expands and contracts with the breath. It is responsible for synchronizing all cells into a shared rhythm that generates a unified identity while it self-soothes. Also known as the energy body, the breath body is activated by

coordinating movement from the breath, which requires the mind to pay attention to the breath. Yoga, tai chi, qi gong, and the martial arts adhere to this basic teaching.

3. Your mind body: This layer of self is home to both your emotions and your thoughts, sandwiched between your intuitive body (the next kosha) and your breath body. The more activated and oxygenated your breath body is, the more attuned you are to the life force. An oxygenated mind is more awake to intuition and generates creative thoughts and positive emotions. The inverse is also true: physical stagnation leads to limited beliefs, thoughts, and emotions.

4. Your intuitive body: Your intuitive body has access to timeless truths and ancestral, nonpersonal wisdom. Accessing this subtle, intelligent layer requires awareness of the present moment. Whereas your mind body can get stuck in the past or the future, your intuitive body is present now. This intuitive layer of the self is most able to perceive an even subtler layer of self—the spirit.

5. Your spirit body: The yogis call this layer the bliss body. Your spirit body is in continuous connection with the most ethereal, profound peace, the ever-ready eternal presence. This body is essence—the furthest from form. This is the essential self—it is beyond words, time, space, and being known. Your spirit body is your personal experience of the unbounded vibration that unceasingly generates the cosmos. When you attend to the deep quiet of spirit, you generate ripples of creativity in your intuitive body, which filters into ideas in your mind body (see Figure 3.2).

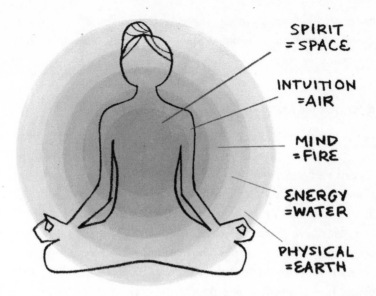

SPIRIT
=SPACE

INTUITION
=AIR

MIND
=FIRE

ENERGY
=WATER

PHYSICAL
=EARTH

Figure 3.2 The koshas and their corresponding elements

Each of your five layers of self is intertwined, married in cause-and-effect patterns, with various needs for development. Each layer can be optimized through specific habits, routines, and rituals.

Simple body habits that nourish and nurture these layers include eating an earlier, lighter dinner; getting to bed early, before 10:00 p.m.; rising and shining early; and drinking enough warm or hot water to stimulate a bowel movement. Tune in to your spirit at dawn by allowing yourself a moment to sit or meditate before your day gets going. Then, move your body—start with ten to twenty minutes of breath-coordinated movement. Plan what, when, and where you'll eat that day while you're tuned in to yourself, ready to start your day, and your bodies are awake. (I'll offer more specific guidance to optimizing each of the bodies in the element chapters in part 2. And if you want a step-by-step guide for the habits of yogis, a few of which were mentioned above, you can find a supportive companion in my first book, *Body Thrive*.)

As better body habits become rituals, your physical body can handle doing more, your mind can learn faster, your intuitive body is more accessible, and you become more receptive to evolutionary growing pains. You'll be less stubborn or reactive when you hit a wall, a break-down before a breakthrough. You'll take time to reflect, receptive to the cyclical nature of growth, opening the door to identity evolution.

5. Heed the Rhythm and the Cycles

Evolution happens in cyclical, informed rhythm. Rhythm is the operating system of evolution, just as our planetary rhythm turns the seasons and diurnal cycles. When you honor rhythms and cycles, you strengthen your cellular memory of natural laws and your cyclical nature, which also empowers your cellular intelligence.

Cycles have parts: the pause, which generates the beginning; the beginning, which generates the maturation; the maturation, which generates the closure; and the closure, which dissolves back into the pause. If you prioritize any part of the cycle over the others, one or more of your bodies takes the hit, lowering your resilience and adaptability. Your intuitive body receives the impulse of the cycles, including the impulse to reflect during the closure part of the cycle. Reflection is notoriously weak in our culture, which prefers to plow ahead at the risk of not learning from yesterday.

Cycles can be short, such as the multiple times per day hunger-satiation cycle, or long, such as the annual cycle of conception, pregnancy, and postpartum. When you align to cycles, you get connected to the cosmos and naturally orient yourself to thrive. For instance, let's look at the hunger-satiation cycle, or the feasting-fasting cycle. Say you overate last night. Today you notice a "residue" in your body and mood, and you have no hunger. If you don't heed the cycle, and you go ahead and eat, you bog down your stomach and intestines. If you heed the cycle, you'll notice an impulse to digest the bog by fasting or exercising. Wait long enough, and you'll notice an *unquestionable* hunger return, completing this hunger-satiation cycle.

Use the next exercise to look for patterns and places for improvement in heeding your cycles. You might notice patterns in honoring cycles that lead to breakthroughs and patterns of habitual breakdowns where your greatest gains can be made.

Find Your Patterns with a Ten-Year Journey Map

This exercise starts with a reflection on cycles, and then you'll sketch your journey map.

Consider: What season are you in now? Are you going toward the dark solstice or the light solstice, the season that brings you inward or outward, respectively? What is the moon phase now, toward fullness or emptiness? If you are menstruating, are you heading toward the extroversion of ovulation or the introversion of menstruation? What phase of life are you in: the growing-up phase, the middle mature-and-creative phase, or the reflective wind-down phase?

Next, you'll sketch a map with colored pens on paper—like a child's treasure map—of your past ten years. (Or, if you prefer, you can journal rather than draw a map.) Reflect on key events, themes, big changes, or chapters. Put your big events, breakdowns, and breakthroughs on your map with any symbols that come to mind. When did you neglect or nourish yourself? Where did you ignore or embrace the cycles? Look for patterns.

On your map or in your journal, include the perspectives of:

- your physical body

- your energy body

- your mind body

- your intuitive body

- your spirit body

Where and when did you heed the cycles? What happened next? Where and when were you out of sync, not listening to your intuitive body? For example, if you had a physical, mental, emotional, or core-relationship breakdown, what preceded it? What were the early signs that you can now see?

In your current journey, what phase of the cycle are you in now? Or are you in that curious pause between cycles, which is also part of the cycle itself, as is the pause between the exhalation and the next inhalation of your breath cycle? Look at your map and the territory you've covered.

Now, draw a map for one year ahead. Start where you are. Listen to all five bodies. Strengthen the part of the cycle that tends to be weakest for you. Perhaps it's the closure, or perhaps it's the pause. Perhaps it's the follow-through or the middle. When you are done, pause. Absorb the power and intelligence in aligning your purpose from the cycles. ■

6. Think Big, Test Small, Fail Fast, Learn Always

Let's say your deeper dream is to be twice as wealthy. You are thinking big in the wealth department. When you think about how to get there, what ideas appear? Make a quick list in your head. Which idea might fly with the least amount of effort? To find out, you might test your idea in a small way.

Say your best idea is investing in a rental property for high-priced weekly rentals. You decide to test your assumptions with a few days of research. You run the numbers on high-end rental investments locally. Your test costs little time or money.

From your research, you learn a few things. Unsexy multifamily housing looks like a better bet—in a region about four hours away. This isn't what you expected. In fact, it's a fast fail for that high-end Airbnb idea. You learned without risk. What new assumptions could you test next? You know time up front saves time later—that's why you are on an iterative cycle of thinking big and testing small for rapid evolution.

This value has its origin in lean startup-and-design thinking: "Think big, test small, fail fast, learn always." *Think big* is your deeper dream. *Test small* is the smallest action you can take to move the needle of progress forward. You're as interested in whether your test fails as you are in whether it succeeds in order to test your assumptions and become better informed. This is the "learn always" part of the equation. This efficient and effective learning feedback loop advances your thinking and ability to see which next small action to test. That small action gives you feedback to incorporate, and naturally you correct your course and test again. You "small test" your deeper dreams into reality.

Rather than getting waylaid in big planning phases, look for small actions to take that test your assumptions. By testing assumptions, we test our beliefs. Often big plans fail because of moving forward too fast without investigating our assumptions. Yet, with this powerful feedback loop, we become more flexible and less defensive about our assumptions and beliefs, which opens us to rapid growth. "Fail fast" gives us permission to experiment without much investment. We want to test our assumptions on our high-impact, low-effort ideas quickly and efficiently, and then move forward.

You can use this acronym, attributed to the eleventh president of India, A. P. J. Abdul Kalam, to reframe failure:[3]

First
Attempt
In
Learning

Failing fast orients us to learning fast and to continual experimentation, the fuel of personal evolution. We become less attached to outcomes and more attached to the *process* that leads to the outcomes—the journey of who we are becoming and the skills, relationships, and competencies required. "Learn always" is the call for reflection, which updates how we think big next. "Learn always" reminds us that with every small, daily experiment in life, our human operating system is built to absorb and integrate new knowledge.

An example of my own experiments with thinking big in terms of peak mental performance was when I tried cryotherapy, or cold therapy. I tested small with a thirty-second cold shower. That was too long, so I dialed it back to ten seconds. From there, I added a few seconds at a time until one minute was easy. Because I was enjoying the anti-inflammatory benefits of the therapy, I wanted to go deeper. I installed a plunge tank in my backyard and quickly realized that sixty degrees was too cold, so I started with ten-second dunks in sixty-five-degree water. A year later, I'm doing ten-minute cold plunges in fifty-five-degree water. Sometimes I plunge in icy creeks in the heart of winter. The improved mental acuity, inflammation-reducing effects, workout recovery benefits, and lymphatic stimulation are tangible, but I had to experiment with incremental changes to get there.

The more you automate the cycle of thinking big, then testing small your assumptions and learning from the outset, the faster and deeper the clarity, knowledge, and momentum you get to experience. In part 2, you'll see this principle in action as you learn the tools to turn your deeper dreams from impossible projects into an exploration with dozens of doable experiments.

7. Invest in You

You are your greatest asset. Your skills, competencies, and even your relationship with yourself are the greatest investments of your time and money because they determine your path and your destination, opening doors to a future better than your past. Yet, in modern culture, the word *invest* most often refers to real estate, insurance, and retirement accounts. This value reconciles how and how much to invest in you.

First, differentiate the word *spend* from the word *invest*. Use *spend* for when you put time, money, or attention into that which has no return or a negative return. Use *invest* for when you put time, money, or attention into something that has a positive return. For example, if you are taking a skill-building course to help you find more interesting work, you are investing in, not spending on, your long-term emotional well-being. Or, if you frequently buy high-quality nutritionally dense nonchemical foods, you can expect a positive return in your physical body, your longevity, and your short-term mental capacity. If you frequently buy low-nutrient, carcinogenic, or processed foods, you incur both short-term and long-term costs to your physical body, your longevity, and your short-term mental capacity. The former is investing; the latter is spending.

This value is a reminder to invest in what makes your heart sing, contributes to your rejuvenation, and enhances your play—all of which decrease later spending on disease care. The adage "all work and no play makes Jack a dull boy" applies here. Treating yourself to what reenergizes you—the people, the retreats, the travel—is an intentional investment that should be guilt free. You will find that the more you attune to this ethic, the more liberated, resilient, and abundant you become.

Invest in You

How does your future self invest? Write a list that reflects your five layers: How does your superheroine invest in her body? Her energy? Her mind? Her intuitive powers? Her spiritual depth? How does your superheroine self invest in her ambition? Her relationships? Who does she invest in for guidance, for support?

First, notice when you use the words *spend, pay,* and *invest.* Use *invest* when you would use *spend* or *pay.* For example, "Pay attention to me!" becomes "Invest your attention in me!" In another example, "I spent $100 on groceries" becomes "I invested $100 to nourish myself." Then, remove *spend* from your vocabulary unless money laid down was not an upgrade with future payback. As you change your language, notice what seems out of integrity. Too many clothes in your closet and stuff in storage has a negative return. That was spending, not investing, behavior.

Reflect on your best investments of time and energy over the past year. Take a moment to realize those investments as seeds for better future investing behavior. ■

8. Embrace a Solid B–

The idea of embracing a B– emerged from breaking the perfectionist mindset with my course members. Growth-oriented people hold high standards for themselves, which can keep them from testing small and failing. Carol Dweck, author and researcher in the field of motivation, identifies perfectionism as "fixed mindset," not "growth mindset." "Fixed mindset" impedes evolution because the emotional body gets flooded with disappointment and disapproval, which triggers a reactionary, regressive response.[4]

If you're a natural risk-taker or experimenter or biohacker who doesn't care much what other people think, then skip onward. But if you're a perfectionist or invest time worrying about how things look from the outside, test this value with a vengeance.

Prioritizing getting it "right" over getting it done can slow your evolution so dramatically that you might regress. You might never finish, publish, or "ship" your project, as they say in tech development, thus weakening the overall, iterative cycle of triumph, completion, and reflection. The details of getting it "right" take too long, and you lose momentum and perspective. You sink your own ship.

But if you give yourself the leeway that comes with embracing a solid B–, you finish! You publish! You ship! Instant feedback from other people—or even, say, the marketplace—efficiently and strategically aligns your next actions. The software development community uses the term *beta phase* when the product contains all of the features and is nearly complete but likely contains known or unknown bugs. Perfectionists: heed the words *cycle, release, beta, bugs, issues, crashes,* and *loss* in the concept of beta testing. Let B– remind you to be better at the beta phase. When you can get 80 percent of the way to your goal, you'll have more than enough momentum, lessons learned, and input to figure out the next best steps.

If you get lost in the details or have a voice that says, "If I can't do it perfectly, I'm not going to do it at all," do the exercise below and come back to this section frequently.

Embrace a Solid B–

Do this exercise as contemplation or by journaling or sketching. Recall a time in your not-so-distant past when you felt like you failed, when you didn't meet your own expectations, but you actually did pretty well. Perhaps you made dinner for some friends, and the food turned out "pretty good." The company was great, but you sabotaged your experience with the label you put on it. Perhaps you planned to run a whole marathon but ended up walking the last ten miles. Perhaps you set a goal of earning 20 percent more income last year and hit 15 percent. Pick any situation in which the idea of what you should have achieved was above and beyond what you actually achieved.

Now, look at the same situation from the B–, or beta, perspective.

What if you required only 80 percent of your desired outcome to feel 100 percent satisfied? Imagine you are 100 percent satisfied with the outcome you actually achieved: the pretty good dinner party, the completed marathon, the 15 percent increase in income.

Now that you're experiencing "enoughness," you set your next goal. Leverage insights from the previous goal in formulating your next goal (learn always). You are on a perpetual growth path. If you want, throw an even more relaxed dinner party. Go from a marathon runner to a marathon speed-walker. Earn more but focus on less effort.

Notice that when you are okay with a B–, or beta phase, experimentation begins. You respond to the creative impulse. You accept and respond to the outcome. You learn and move forward. In chapter 7, we'll expand on this value in working with air element. ■

9. Trust Your Desire

Your deeper dreams trust your desire. Desire is intrinsically intelligent and bigger than you. It's divine—the way spirit directs you to make something happen in your life. Desire speaks when you find the juice, the flow, the nectar, the joy. Desire is embedded in your identity evolution, your five bodies, and your heeding the cycles. If you diminish desire, you eclipse the light of your spirit body, overriding the informed impulses of your intuitive body. Often, you need to shift from thinking to feeling what the physical body, energy body, or spirit body desires. If you don't trust desire, you diminish your life force and thus your life.

When you think big, big desires arise. For example, if you're deeply exhausted, your big desire is to rest. You might think, *Sounds nice, but who is going to do the dishes?* Some of us are so tired that the simple rituals of daily living, such as doing the dishes, the closure cycle of a good meal, no longer bring joy. Overriding rest weakens you at your core and sets up your body for disease, from mono to chronic fatigue syndrome. The pattern that led to exhaustion—overspending energy rather than investing in rejuvenation—might seem impossible to change. When you don't slow down to be present for the simple rituals of returning objects to their places in your home, bathing, cooking, or tending children, life itself becomes a joyless burden. To reconnect with desire, revive joy, and restore rhythm, honor the feel-good intelligence of rest. Think big and test small with the pleasures of what truly nourishes and nurtures you. We'll explore this process thoroughly in chapter 5, on earth element.

Small actions build immune resilience. Your deep dreams will stir. Then, you'll notice you are heeding the rhythm and nurturing all five bodies. You'll see how all the values connect and orient you back to your center. As you become well rested, game on. You'll unlock new levels of trusting your desire. Begin with small actions in trusting your body, your energy, your intuition, and your uplifting relationships. You'll move on to trusting how you design your space (see chapter 4) and how you own your time (see chapter 7). Eventually you'll trust life and the cosmos and appreciate all four parts of the cycles of evolution.

Trust Your Desire

Consider the day ahead or tomorrow. How does your physical body want to feel? Do a body check-in. You can quickly pass your hands over your skin or clothes to feel your bodies. How does your spirit body want to feel tomorrow? As you collect your intelligence, park your judgment and mental chatter in the corner. Do you want to feel heavier or lighter? More grounded or freer? Hot or cold? Have more movement or more rest? More activity or more relaxation? What is present? Design tomorrow for that.

Now, if your bossy mind says you need intense exercise, but your physical body screams for rest and nourishment, park your mind. Design tomorrow to recover your body's joy. It's just one small experiment to vitalize your ability to dream big.

We'll plunge deeper into how to empower desire's intelligence while navigating challenging terrain in chapter 8, on water element. ∎

10. Leverage Your Strengths

You are unique. You have natural advantages to escort your potential into reality. Kristen Wheeler, founder of nativegenius.com, calls these advantages your native genius: "It's unique intelligence that's innate to you. It arises naturally—it's not manufactured or acquired. When cultivated, it has the potential to be exceptional."[5] Native genius is an asset—a key strength to leverage.

Your natural way of being, when employed consciously, becomes a strength, and you can leverage your strengths intentionally. You can determine how your puzzle pieces fit into your deeper dreams and what intrinsic advantages you possess to realize your next chapter of becoming. For instance, if you are meticulous and detail-oriented and have good follow-through, these are assets. Your care and conscientiousness lead you to finish what you start. You likely don't jump into things but rather carefully assess where to direct your energy. Your downfall might be trading the big picture and the time line for the details. Paired with passionate visionaries, creators, or innovators who might move too fast for their own good, you can provide guardrails and generate a solid system for their ideas to come to fruition. The big idea moves forward, and details are assessed based on necessity at that stage.

To find your native strengths, take personality and cognitive tests such as:

- Wealth Dynamics

- How to Fascinate

- Gallup Strengths Finder

- DISC Profile

- KOLBE Index

Through these tests, you will know and be able to communicate your strengths and learn which kinds of partners complement you. To leverage your strengths, repeat this cycle:

- Know specifically what your strengths are right now.

- Communicate them accurately and easily.

- Develop them strategically.

- Find counterparts with opposite strengths—you need each other.

When I took the tests mentioned above, according to Wealth Dynamics I'm a "creator" and a "star." This lined up with How to Fascinate, which labeled me an "avant-garde" (a combination of innovation and prestige). In the Gallup Strengths Finder, I'm strong in focus and command, and I'm an "activator, futurist, and achiever." Together, these tests inform me that my native genius, or clear advantage, is in innovating and influencing others to take part. From the DISC Profile, I know I have quick-start energy, and follow-through isn't my strength. Therefore, it's imperative that I find and nurture partnerships with counterparts who are good with details, excel at maintaining systems, and naturally set guardrails around the fast-moving train.

After you take a few personality and cognitive tests, you will see the strengths you have to leverage.

Leverage Your Strengths

Take at least two of the five tests listed above or reference those you've already taken. Each test has a unique angle or viewpoint.

The combination of test results will point to your native genius, your unique innate intelligence. We're all geniuses, especially when we cultivate our natural proclivities. Invest in you by investing in the tests.

Next, leverage your investment. After you recognize your natural strengths, communicate your strengths to others. Articulate your unique genius in a few words. You can use this sentence stem: "I've recently discovered I have a natural strength in _____. How do you see this in me?" Talk about your strengths. Ask the people close to you what your strengths are and how those strengths are an asset to them. Be available to talk about their intrinsic strengths. See what arises. In chapter 6, on fire element, we'll rely in part on your personality test results and these conversations. ■

11. Learn. Mentor. Master. Cocreate.

We rise and fall together. The best way to learn is to teach. These aphorisms reflect the power of the mentoring relationship. From the strengths you identified, you'll see opportunities to be a mentor or leader to people who need those strengths to realize their deeper dreams. The best way to master something is to teach someone else. It's how we discover what we really know . . . and what we don't. As you mentor, you master. Through mentoring someone in even something as simple as how to cook a soup, build a budget spreadsheet, or manage a project, you become an asset to other people's deeper dreams. The cycle repeats and grows, leading to exponential possibilities.

It's not *all* sunshine and roses, of course. Although learning might seem relatively easy, any degree of mastery requires grit and perseverance. Mentoring develops mastery. Mentoring takes us into the realm of other people, which can get messy and complicated. If your strengths are people-oriented, or relational, this comes more easily to you. If your strengths are task-oriented, or project-focused, this might be a skill to develop.

This value suggests scouting out mentors. Develop and nurture long-term relationships with people who have strengths or mastery in areas that could help you. Think of a community's potential if it would emphasize learning, mentoring, and mastering. As you build relationships, you build tensile strength around your ambitions. Sense your potential for cocreativity—where could your ambitions interconnect with teamwork? Where would a mentor or master be helpful? And how does your native genius point you toward mentoring others? You might notice that cocreating leads to next-level potential for collective evolution and leadership.

Learn. Mentor. Master. Cocreate.

A powerful catalyst for recognizing the importance of mentoring is writing and sending a letter. Letter writing is a reflective process that activates the power of gratitude, awakening your intuition and your spirit for your dharma.

Recognize a master who has mentored you—whether at work, at school, in the kitchen (it might be your mother), or in the workshop (it might be your uncle). You can even write a letter to someone who has passed—the effect will not be lost. Write by hand from your heart, and express what you learned from them. Your letter can be very short. Openly revere that powerful soul for what value they delivered to your life. As you do, you bestir the power of our ancient human mentoring relationship. You might choose to keep the letter private, or you can send the letter to them or their children, which will light up their spirits.

Next, consider someone you have mentored, in any capacity, however informally, at any time in your life, and write a letter to them too. Let them know the growth you have seen. Perhaps recall their desires and their struggles. You might even express appreciation for them taking action to reach their goals.

After you have written the two letters, pause. This is the closure part of heeding the learning, mentoring, mastering, and cocreating cycle. Notice the reverberations from these two relationships. Notice the cycle of learn, mentor, master, cocreate. After a few iterations, you can mentor your kid or your friend through the entire Master of You process. ■

12. Shift from Consumer to Collaborator

The early etymological root of the word *consumer* is "squanderer." The word *consumer* has two modern shoots: economics and ecology. In the economy, the consumer pays to use a product or experience a service. In ecology, a consumer is a being that eats another being.

Seeing a consumer as a squanderer can be deeply disturbing and, in a word, explain planetary exploitation. When we shift to being conscious collaborators rather than consumers, we activate the values of respect, cooperation, and teamwork.

The rise of the internet and social media created tools and platforms for people to express and advocate for what they truly value. A 2010 *Forbes* article reported the shift in the marketplace from people being passive *con*sumers to influential *pro*sumers—advocates of what they wanted to promote—and successful companies were paying attention to what *pro*sumers were saying about them.[6] The article then offered suggestions to help businesses adapt to the evolving marketplace, encouraging them to "join the conversation" and "develop relationships with those people by interacting with them, providing useful information, and being accessible and human." Smarter businesses collaborate with their customers, just as smart farmers collaborate with the ecosystem they are farming.

This shift to prosumer is the beginning of the revolution from consumer to collaborator. The one-way street is becoming a two-way relationship, creating the ability to collaborate on mutual desires. There is a flow of energy and intelligence regarding the goods and services, however gross or subtle, people exchange. We shift from unconscious squanderer to conscious cocreator, placing the collaborator—the person investing time, energy, or currency—at center stage.

When we shift from consumer to collaborator, we activate our interconnectedness. This interconnectedness has been called the *web of life*. This mindset—being part of something larger—enlivens and renews us with a sense of being supported, being simultaneously part of a larger whole and an activator within the web. Our soul is not just intelligent, it's intertelligent —it has the ability to access the larger wisdom of the web of life.

For example, I apply this value to what I watch on the big screen. If the characters aren't inspiring, learning, and growing, I'm not going to squander my time. However, if I love it or learn from it, I'll activate the web through the power of my voice within my community. Now I'm a prosumer—an advocate—an influencer. I'm collaborating through feedback. When you stop consuming what is mediocre by being more selective with your attention, your appreciation, your voice, and your social currency, you advance the conversation of which you are a part. By vocalizing desire, your voice influences the marketplace. You shift from victim to activator, cocreating our future. As a collaborator, you spread what you value.

Collaborate with What You Consume

PART 1: FOOD

On the most primitive level and on the physical body level, we rely on ecosystems for food. To shift from a consumer of food to a collaborator with food, consider having a conversation with food. You can start with the food in your natural foods market or the food in your fridge. This conversation can be silent.

It might go something like this, "Hello, apple. Where were you grown? What can I do to support the tree you came from?"

Or when you enter the produce aisle, ask the fruit and vegetables, "Who wants to come home with me?" Then pause. Listen from your intuitive body. Leave the mind body out of it! Dare to fail, to learn, to connect with the intelligence of the life force in the produce aisle. Notice what you put into your cart, which will later feed your cells, become your tissue, and activate your deeper dreams into reality.

PART 2: BOOK

Recall the last book you read that you loved. If you loved it, how did it serve you—through the ideas, the art, the characters, or the ethos of the book? What does it cultivate or perpetuate that you want to see more of in tomorrow's world? What could you do to collaborate with the author or the book itself? Write a quick list of small actions (in other words, test small) that you could take to activate the power of that book.

From easy to hard, here are a few ideas: You could mention it to a friend today. You could write a review on Amazon. You could share a quote on social media. You could message the author. You could recommend it to your local library for purchase. You could do a book club with a few friends.

Notice how just from making a list, you are collaborating with the book and the author. By generating the next stage of the conversation, you vote for tomorrow's world. ■

When your actions are in line with your values, you are attuned to your higher purpose. In the words of *Atomic Habits* author James Clear, "Every action you take is a vote for the type of person you wish to become. No single instance will transform your beliefs, but as the votes build up, so does the evidence of your new identity."[7] If you find daily opportunities to practice the Master of You ethos, it will be easier to step into your next purpose and projects.

Start to notice the ethos at work. Notice if you catch yourself spending on or consuming something in which you don't want to invest. If you're a reforming perfectionist, you might see how you set yourself up for drudgery by aiming for an A+ rather than taking quicker actions to get to a B–. Notice where you can reflect on your strengths and bring up your native genius in conversation. Notice how your unique strengths are an asset to your deeper dreams. Notice your cycles—with fatigue, with hunger, with the beginning and end of the day—and how they fit into the larger, delightful cycles of rejuvenation and nourishment.

Throughout this book, we'll practice these twelve values. Articulating your ethos makes it identifiable and communicable. And having shared values leads you to natural partnerships and collaborations with people by whom your deeper dreams can be fueled and informed. You'll also notice that with this ethos, your choices consistently come from a place of integrity, and you stretch into previously uncharted realms that come with growth and depth. Ethical alignment paves the way for honest, compelling relationships and faster growth. You might notice that you clarify your language to articulate what you mean, that you uplevel the bar for those in whom you want to invest your time, and that you set yourself up for satisfying days and a life that leaves a legacy of dignity and delight.

Now you understand the mindset, the ethos operating system, underlying *Master of You*. Let's harness the elements.

PART II

Master Your Five Elements

You've laid groundwork in part 1 to unearth and breathe new life into your deeper dreams and your next dharma. You awakened your next purpose and became familiar with the elements (see Figure P1) and an ethos to align and support all of your ambitions. You are solidly on the ladder of your next self-invention. Next, you'll immerse yourself in the hidden powers within each element, which you will unleash in pursuit of living your next potential, leaving no part of yourself behind.

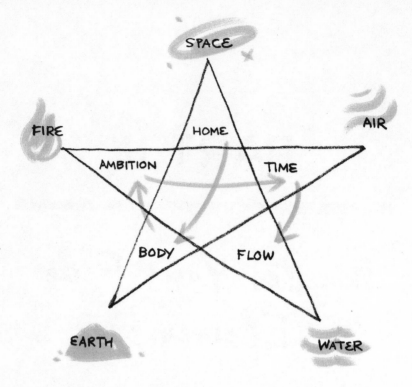

Figure P1 The five-pointed star shows the relationship of the five dynamic elements and our directional path through the Master of You process. Space, the lightest, is on top, and the weightier elements are on the bottom, with the dynamic elements flanking the sides.

In the next five chapters, you will become intimate with the elements, starting with space, characterized by your spirit, your home, and your workplace. Space is the easiest place to start and the easiest element to return to whenever you run into roadblocks along the way through the elements. There is no rush up the elemental ladder to the next version of yourself. Going slowly through the elements leads to unexpected accelerations down the road. Remember this as you traverse the next five chapters. You are escorting your deeper dreams into reality. Master of You is an iterative process; the more you apply it, season by season, the more you find you are living a deeply aligned life.

4

SPACE: MASTER OF HOME

astering space is intentionally refining your home and work environments. Your goal in this chapter is to restructure the spaces in which you live and work to call forth and nurture your next self along the trajectory of your identity evolution, with ease and efficiency. You will upgrade your environments—where you live, where you work, where you rejuvenate, and where you prepare your food—to help you select the habits and experience the feelings that lead you to your next superheroine (or superhero) self.

In mastering space, you consciously arrange space to create an inspired environment. The Sanskrit word *akasha* translates to "the home for all objects in the universe," or the ether element, space. Akasha is all-enclosing, all-pervading, omnipotent, omniscient, and omnipresent. It's the first expression of consciousness coming into form, all the space in the expanding cosmos.[1] Space has no resistance and, therefore, complete freedom. Space inspires the freedom within us to create and re-create ourselves. The easiest and most accessible frontier is how we shape the spaces we inhabit, with the intention of reshaping ourselves.

In this chapter, you'll intentionally design your spaces to resonate with five words that best serve your deeper dreams. You'll call forth the superheroine or superhero you created in chapter 3 to sort your stuff. In the process, you'll digest who you have been, allowing your past identities to integrate and then steer you toward an even brighter future, one in which you will be more capable and confident knowing who you've been and who you are becoming.

If you're thinking, *All that sounds dandy, but I share my spaces with other people and their stuff,* don't worry, I've got your back. You'll get a primer on how to upgrade shared spaces based on your common values to get the people in your life onboard. Last, you'll learn a practice to settle into your emerging identity that will keep you from slipping into outdated habits and identities.

YOUR SPACE INFLUENCES YOUR THOUGHTS, HABITS, AND IDENTITY

Have you ever walked into a space—a home, an office, a garden, a building—that instantly elevated your mood and your thinking? Recall the space that inspired you, in which you felt called to be your best self—the lighting, the airflow, and the proportion of space and objects mindfully placed that enhanced the room. Such spaces invite you to be uniquely you, inspiring the feeling that you can do anything you set your mind to. Spaces can uplift you to be a better version of yourself and trigger those next-level thoughts and choices.

The spaces we create at home, at work, and in the car predispose us to specific habits and reinforce beliefs, values, cravings, thoughts, and even our orientation toward stress or ease. Our spaces trigger habits that orient our trajectory toward either radiant longevity or premature aging. Your living and working spaces influence your thoughts and ideas, which arise and are impressed upon the inner space of your emotional and intuitive bodies (koshas).

Benjamin Hardy, a self-improvement thought leader and author of *Willpower Doesn't Work*, places priority on environment: "The next evolution of high performance and achievement takes the focus off the individual and places the environment at the forefront. Thus, ironically, the future of self-help will not be focused on 'the self,' but rather, it will be focused on the environment that shapes the self. At the core of this new thrust will be the installment of enriched environments."[2] Your ambitions require a refined environment that preselects specific small daily habits, beliefs, thoughts, and relationships. You redesign your spaces to support your ambitions to birth your next identity.

When your living spaces become clutter-free oases (including inside your drawers, closets, and storage areas), your inner space effortlessly attunes to the frequency of your potential. Ayurveda explains this experience as *svastha*, which means "seated in the self," and it is a crucial component in the definition of health. When you are seated in yourself, your spirit is embedded and embodied in your cells; this is a prerequisite to thriving. In svastha, you are rooted and whole, able to be present, reflective, and innovative. Design your spaces for svastha.

By purposefully restructuring your environments, you actively process your past identities. Your past patterns surface as beliefs, assumptions, and thoughts. As you digest your past, you upgrade your spaces and summon the experience of akasha, with the freedom to become greater than who you've been. When you are inspired, supported, and undistracted from within, you catch glimpses, visions, of your next dharma and the identity that supports that dharma.

Vibrations

The elements are best understood with conceptual thinking, which is symbolic and experiential, rather than with rational, linear thinking. Space is the subtlest element, the hardest to grasp; it is the concept of potentiality and emptiness at the same time, expanding in a nonlinear way, unbound by time. Space emerges first in the elemental progression of essence to form, potential to matter, subtle to gross, and impulse to action. Space is full of vibrations.

You have probably noticed how the space in a forest or a sacred temple or church *feels* different from that of a messy bathroom or a dive bar. Inventor and futurist Nikola Tesla articulated this universal concept in the early 1900s when he reportedly said, "If you want to find the secrets to the universe think of energy, frequency and vibration."[3] Vibrations can range from low frequency to high frequency, from those in a void or vacuum to those in a highly charged space, from emotionally uplifting to depressing, from scattered to rooted.

Space also defines the vibratory atmosphere within your cells. Space is the subtle realm of feelings, sensations, and intuition. For us supersentient humans, vibrations become tangible as feelings, thoughts, and ideas. We then manifest our words and actions from our emotions and thoughts. Space resonates with possibility, potentiality, malleability, and mindful presence, giving masters of space the power to manifest more with less effort. Yet, in modern culture, we overcrowd our schedules, our homes, our minds, and even our stomachs. We sacrifice ease when we sacrifice space.

The Sanskrit words *sukha* and *dukkha* are etymologically related to akasha—the ether element. Akasha is the subtlest of the elements, and because of that, it is most easily influenced by positive or negative vibrations. Sukha, or clean space, carries the pure vibration and intelligence of the life force. When you are in a sukha environment—perhaps a temple, a pristine forest, or a clean kitchen, you can feel how the life force flows through it. When you are in a dukkha environment, or dirty space, perhaps a disheveled basement or garage, the dust and jumbled objects are blocking the flow of the life force by diminishing the vibration of pure space.

Gauging sukha and dukkha can be very helpful in the process of aligning your spaces to your dharma. In ancient times, dukkha was associated with malignant purpose and violence to the self. This implies that maligned space harms our ability to perceive the subtle signals of dharma. Unoptimized space generates unnecessary stress and feelings of deprivation and dissatisfaction.

In the body, dukkha deteriorates into pain, addiction, and disease, whereas sukha generates lasting happiness and integrated health. In the same way, disorganized or disharmonic spaces violate, rather than support, your dharma, causing you to lose energy, health, and momentum. Notably, one of the definitions of dharma is to uphold what is good, true, and beautiful. Disorganization in your fridge, in your drawers, on your counters, or on your desk disrupts you in navigating your life effectively. Disharmonic space muffles your intuition, scatters your mind, and overwhelms your emotions, which ultimately obscures your dharma. For your superheroine self to gain traction, you'll declutter and reinvigorate your spaces to uphold your clear, aligned purpose.

To master your spaces, you'll sort your stuff to find out which possessions uphold your next dharma. Sorting presses your reset button and refreshes your spirit with the frequency of possibility. Like defragmentation of a computer, sorting speeds up your household and work operating systems. If you structure all of your spaces, from your closet to your kitchen to your bathroom drawers, you can prioritize the habits and the feelings your superheroine wants. Redesigning your space to reduce the drag of outdated patterns invigorates the person you are becoming. Ultimately, you separate wheat from chaff—your future from your past, your possessions from your donations.

To separate requires *viveka*, the Sanskrit concept of discernment, used in yoga. With discernment you differentiate, without attachment, outdated patterns from potential, liberating stuck energy into motion. In yoga philosophy, viveka is often paired with *vairagya*, which means freedom from attachment. With practice, you will easily and honestly distinguish what generates flow from what reverberates drag. Initially, you might cling to your familiar and comfortable stuff as well as the patterns the stuff reinforces. Vairagya reminds you to let go of your stuff and the patterns of your past. You are bigger than the "you" you were. A future self is emerging, with new needs. These two powers—to differentiate (viveka) and to release dispassionately (vairagya)—set you free to become more authentic, honest, integrated, powerful, and wise. Now it's time to re-create your home, office, car, wardrobe, bathroom, kitchen, refrigerator, and storage with the Five Words Exercise.

Five Words

How do you feel in your space? Do you spend time looking for things? Do you wear most of the things in your closet or drawers—or are they full of who knows what? Does your bathroom inspire your daily pampering? Does your fridge make it easy to select fresh vegetables? Does your office help you think clearly? Does your garage contain your favorite toys and tools, not a bunch of other stuff?

Here is a simple exercise to recalibrate your space:

1. Recall the particulars of your deeper dreams and the person that you want to become to achieve that. What does the home, the office, the fridge, and the bathroom of that person look like?

2. Ask yourself, your superheroine: What is the frequency or feeling that you want to create? How do you want your space to feel? How do you want your space to look? What do you want your space to do for you?

3. Choose five adjectives—the five words—that are the most vibrant and true. Words that course members have used include vibrant, fun, playful, sweet, luscious, holistic, bright, purposeful, rooted, inspirational, empowering, joyful, gorgeous, modern, and nurturing.

4. Your five words should describe the qualities of the space in which you want to bathe your cells. Write all of the five words on multiple sticky notes. Put these notes where you'll notice them—your bathroom mirror, your laptop cover, your fridge.

That's it. Now your superheroine knows the calibration you want. These five words will come in handy again, so be sure to find the right words before proceeding.

For example, as Cate, the Legendary Leader (which sounds oh-so-egoic, and yours should too!), my five specific qualities are:

1. modern

2. useful

3. stylish

4. spacious

5. communal

I, along with my family, have received, recorded, and revisited these words when making all decisions about what stays or leaves our home as well as how our possessions are organized to guide our lived experience. If you, too, cohabitate, choose your five words both independently, for your private spaces, and with the other members of your home or office for your shared spaces.

When you're re-forming the unreal into the real, chaos into the known, your words shape what happens next. ■

Master Your Constitution: Learn the Doshas

Recall your constitution from chapter 2. Because the doshas are forces (like verbs), each element creates unique opportunities for each constitutional type. In each element chapter, I offer specific advice for each constitution in a sidebar like this one.

In terms of space, vata types can ground their airy nature by sheltering themselves with a comfy and creative home and office to soften their edges and invite relaxation with warm colors and fabrics. Kapha types should design an airy, more modern, minimalist home and office—spaces that feel expansive, organized, and energized with bright colors. Pittas thrive in a clean, calm home and office with plants and cooling colors.

YOUR SUPERHEROINE SORTS YOUR STUFF

Fascinatingly, you won't employ accurate viveka (discernment) with your stuff in its current resting place. Your stuff is associated with that place, giving it a sticky advantage over your emotions. You need to move it out, expose it to the light of day, and let your dharma decide:

uphold or release. Tap into your superheroine self to sort your stuff based on upholding your five words, according to those vibrations. Intuit your superheroine's personality, her habits, and her desires to differentiate what you keep and what you let go. By the end of the sorting process, you'll find a set point, with everything you keep located in its new special spot.

Marie Kondo, the guru of tidying up, advises sorting your stuff by categories, not by rooms. Kondo's evolutionary sequence of sorting begins with clothing, then books, papers, dishes, furniture, and finally memorabilia. She begins with the stuff physically closest to your heart (your clothes, beginning with your shirts and jackets), then moves sequentially to the more mundane, and then finally addresses your etheric heartstrings—the memories you choose to keep. You reshape yourself by sorting past identities, from your wardrobe to your mementos.[4] When you sort your stuff in this way, you are actually processing the emotions associated with the memories attached to each item.

As you're sorting, you might notice that special items emerge from all categories as memorabilia—items that hold special meaning, value, and significance beyond their utility. This process of honoring your past, including items from your ancestors, helps you digest memories and attributes of your ancestors you want to uphold, while releasing the energy of bad memories or disharmonies from your past selves. For example, my friend Elise, author of *SuperAger*, holds on to a 1940s ribbon-knit dress from her grandmother, who was exactly her size. The ribbon dress reminds Elise of their shared value of femininity, which Elise didn't get from her own mother. Yet, Elise recycled a photo collection of herself that her grandmother assembled for her only granddaughter, with photos that reflected a person Elise never felt inside that she was.

Another Master of You course member in the process of minimizing her possessions decided she would sell her condo and live abroad. When paring down her stuff, she had a strong urge to destroy ten years' worth of journals and letters. "These journals I wrote on my path to sobriety; the letters I received in support. I've been sober for years, and I want to burn them." She loved the suggestion to schedule a ritual to mark the end of this chapter of her life and invite those who supported her to participate or to send a note reflecting who she has become in their eyes. She feels immeasurably liberated from the weight of her past as she explores her next dharma.

To get yourself started, reserve time to go through just one category at a time. You'll gain momentum after you get started. You'll feel a difference in your space immediately. Each category might take half a day, a day, a weekend, or a week, depending on how much you have and how quickly you sort. When you complete your clothes, move on to books, then papers, then dishes, décor, office supplies, hobby stuff, maintenance supplies, and finally sentimental items. The first time you do this takes the longest.

You will eventually sort through all you own. Each object in your possession has a current essence, a presence, a vibration. Recall your super-heroine self and your five words. As you are deciding whether an object stays or goes, feel for a "Hell, yeah!" What doesn't match the higher frequency goes. Use this discernment with every item under your care. Make this your chief obsession, *sadhana* (spiritual practice), and form of entertainment until you are done. My advice is to get it done within one month, one moon cycle, using whatever crevice of time available. Lengthening it will drag your dharma backward. If you cohabitate, get your housemates onboard (I have some suggestions for doing so below). It's contagious. You'll eventually develop a natural, seasonal rhythm, making mastering space fun and easy.

Note that most people overestimate the "value" of their possessions. I recommend letting go to move forward. This process cures you of buying excessively, meaning you'll invest smarter in the long run, so get your stuff out fast. Rather than trying to squeeze money out of your belongings from reselling them, donate your stuff to let it live out its next purpose. However, for monetarily valuable items, you'll make more money in less time selling on Facebook, eBay, or in consignment stores than having a garage or estate sale.

SHARED SPACES AND COMMON VALUES

If you share your living or working space, you likely notice how the communal space steers you all toward particular experiences, certain emotions, and predictable habits. Most Master of You course members unwittingly find themselves in the role of leader of their cohabitants. Because you picked up this book, chances are you will also need to take the lead in your communal spaces. To avoid your cohabitants seeing this as yet another self-improvement plan that you're thrusting upon them (which might be true), look for natural and informal ways to get the people in your life in touch with their superhero (using the exercise in chapter 3). Be mindful of the challenging nature of this process. Get people thinking about their unique five words before collectively coming up with five words for your communal spaces and diving into sorting together. Do this seasonally, and you'll find that mastering space together becomes natural.

Tips for Sorting Your Stuff with the People in Your Life

- Remind yourselves of your shared values and discuss how your communal space could better reflect your values this season.

- Together, find five words for your collective space using the Five Words Exercise.

- Post those words publicly—on the fridge or a chalkboard—to guide the process.

- Make a schedule for sorting your communal stuff together, and stick to it.

- With your children, partner, or elders, guide them into sorting their personal things on a schedule, without your input in the actual sorting, and without disempowering them by doing it for them.

This process might stir latent issues, some of which might have been hidden under the rug for a while. Before you begin, make sure you've identified your shared values in a list (refer to chapter 3). You can usually do this quite quickly and then use it as a reference to remind you of your collective ethos. As an example, in our home, part of our value code is embedded in the sentence, "Everything has one place, and there's one place for everything." As a result, we don't spend time hunting down possessions. We also have values around pitching in to keep our communal space neat, clean, and in good condition. My daughter has trained her friends to clean up before moving on to the next activity, whether that's making a meal or doing an art project. It's part of our ethos and our house rules. We all agreed this is how we want our space to feel, so we uphold this value with our habits.

Sometimes cohabitants uncover a big rift in their ethos or in how they want to shape their space. If this happens, read chapter 3 together, and look for any common ground in the values. For example, you might agree that "orienting yourselves to thrive" is a good idea. Discuss what this means and how each person can shape the shared space to reinforce their own thriving—in their body, in their work, and in their relationships. Seek common ground, appreciate resonance, and aim for a solid B–, with small tests to learn always. If, in this process, you don't find common ground with any of the twelve values, you might need to seek counseling, individually or together. Know that as painful as it might be to unearth your dreams and discover big rifts, and as difficult as the conversations might be, you're integrating yourself and your space. You will find your common ground.

DIGEST YOUR PAST IDENTITIES

As behavioral researcher Benjamin Hardy reflects, "You and your environment are extensions of each other."[5] As you sort your stuff, emotions get stirred up because your self needs to digest your past. You're processing the emotions—the feelings and lessons learned—of your past identities, digesting on a material level who you have been. Raw emotions might surface in all varieties, requiring your conscious presence to release them. In Ayurveda, emotional *ama*, or unprocessed emotions, act like a dysfunctional residue (just like physical ama in the body, as discussed in the next chapter), blocking the potential for more positive vibrations. In sorting your stuff, you detoxify your emotional body by processing the memories that get stirred up by objects. Detox is always assisted by self-compassion and nurturing. Nurture yourself through this process by eating light nutritious meals, taking baths, taking walks or short meditation breaks, and going to bed early. Bodywork and counseling can also help. The process of sorting possessions encourages communication between your heart and your mind. Appreciate your efforts to recalibrate your space to hear and heed your spirit. As you evolve your space, you evolve your self. Your body will continue to detox emotionally and physically. Use the next exercise to engage this process of letting go of outdated patterns.

Expand Your Inner Space

Each day your body and mind take in more experiences. This accumulation of impressions, emotions, thoughts, and memories is balanced by short periods of emptying out the thoughts and emotions and refreshing your body with breath. This is where the practice of *pranayama*, or the art of breathing, comes in handy. The yogis have used the practice of pranayama for a few millennia to awaken and lighten up the subtle body.

Breathing to expand your inner space is a time-tested method to open your mind through the power of your lungs and also "declutters" your cells.

1. Sit in a comfortable position with your spine lifted and long. Exhale by emptying your lungs slowly, just like you emptied your home of excess stuff. You are making space by emptying out before you take in more. Allow the in-breath to fill your lungs.

2. Pause. Experience this fullness of breath. Now, use your breathing muscles to empty it. Explore. What muscles does this inner space excavation awaken? Use them. They are all yours. Pause in this emptiness. Notice that you have a number of muscles—all sorts of abs and intercostals—that work together with the diaphragm. You're getting a subtle body workout, exercise for your breathing apparatus.

3. Repeat a few cycles. You just did some inner body space clearing. Can you feel your cells circulating the *prana*, the life force, you inhaled? Repeat daily, even if just for a moment or two. Hook this practice to your before-bed routine, or even do it in bed before sleep.

As a result of doing this exercise regularly, you will notice you have an easier time letting go of outdated habits. You are breathing space and life into your cells, supporting the release of past identities and the stale habits that sustained them. You might notice small improvements in your body habits, and even in how you speak, what you say, and your overall attitude. ■

FROM CONSUMER TO COLLABORATOR

Remember, you are developing your yogic superhero powers of viveka (discernment) and vairagya (letting go). As you strengthen these skills, like the force in Luke Skywalker and Princess Leia, your superheroine identity becomes tangible. If at first you don't trust your power to discriminate between your possessions wisely and let go of some, don't fret. With practice, you develop an intuitive trust. You are shifting your identity from a static person (a noun) into a more dynamic human being (a verb). Soon your space will resonate at the frequency of your five words, and it will be highly adaptable if those words change. In this process, you'll notice three things:

1. Less is more until you find your set point. Just enough of the right stuff gives the qualities you want in your space and the experience of freedom, clear thinking, and mastery over your time. (We'll unpack the time component in chapter 7, on air element.)

2. You care for the possessions you keep. Because you have less stuff, and it has a higher resonance, you'll appreciate and take better care of your possessions. You'll treasure your treasures.

3. What you keep deserves a special spot. Now you have less stuff that is more valuable to you, giving your space the frequency you want. As my family says, "Everything has one place, and there's one place for every thing." Put objects in places to prioritize certain habits—this is as simple as refreshing your movement or meditation space, placing fresh-cut vegetables on the side door of your fridge, and placing only the one book you want to read on the coffee table. Collaborate with your stuff to help it find its new home. You'll shift from a consumer of stuff to a collaborator with spaces. This is mastery of space.

Seasonally, you'll feel pulled to update your spaces to meet your emergent needs. You'll notice that this practice becomes a go-to habit when you want to find your center. Mastering space becomes a natural way to collaborate with your evolving dharma.

As you master space through the processes of sorting and letting go, you birth your next set point, which occurs when the space you have cultivated resonates with your deeper dreams. You'll know when you've reached your set point because your space will feel very "awake," as if it's pulling forward a better version of you. You will feel uplifted and inspired in your home, office, car, or whatever space you inhabit; your environment will be an active tool to steer you toward better habits. The late Buddhist and yoga teacher Michael Stone, in his enlivening TEDx Talk "A Deeper Materialism," teaches that rather than using our spiritual practice for the "vertical" transcendence of escape, we should point our attention to the "horizontal" transcendence of connecting through relationship. Our relationships to each other and to everything in our lives are the keys to what he calls "deeper materialism."[6] When we care for and collaborate with our private space, we naturally do the same with public spaces. Stone says, "We are not materialistic enough. Being materialistic means loving the material. It means loving our sidewalks, our lakes, our inventions, our technology, the kind of buildings we move around in, the kind of communities we want to grow."[7] After you've sorted your spaces, and you have only what you can truly care for, notice how your spaces nurture and inspire you.

UPGRADE RESONANCE IN YOUR OUTER SPACE AND INNER SPACE

After you've sorted your stuff, soak in your space. Feel the passing of time. Notice your emotions and thought patterns. You are bathing in your own vibration. Your space is working for you instead of you working on your space. This is what it feels like to have aligned space.

When you've removed the stuff that caused dissonance in your space, distraction in your mind, and busyness in your day, you'll notice more refined levels of resonance. Resonance is when one object vibrating at the same natural frequency of a second object forces that second object into the same vibrational motion. You may have heard of the grandfather clock synchronizing all the clocks in the shop. Synchronization is possible because the clocks' pendulums swing at the same natural frequency. Resonance happens when one object can't help but influence the vibrational frequency of a second object.[8] Resonance will happen when your space reflects your dreams—when they have the same natural vibrational frequency. And you will attune to the vibrations in your space in the same way a smaller clock attunes to the grandfather clock.

With resonance, you unlock the experience of *sthira*, or stillness. Sthira encompasses the experience of cosmic order, of deep peace. Sthira accompanies sukha, or clean space. With the right amount of the right stuff in the right place, your inner stillness thrives. After you bring about sukha and sthira, your sense of time will expand, unlocking present-moment awareness and mental clarity. With more awareness and mental clarity, fire element comes into play, sharpening your focus on your future. Later, you'll need this visionary focus to strategize an effective plan to achieve your ambitions and live your dharma at the next level.

ARCHITECT YOUR ATMOSPHERE

In the process of restructuring your environment, you naturally prioritized the smarter habits of your superheroine self, freeing you from the inefficiency of decision fatigue. Decision fatigue happens after many choices have been made in a row and results in a deteriorated quality of decision making, when your willpower fails, often because of a dukkha environment or one that reinforces outdated and unwanted habits. As a result, you have been in an endless cycle of identity stagnation. By the end of the day, it's nearly impossible to make smart choices about what to eat, how to unwind the mind and move the body, how to reflect on the day and power down, and when to go to bed. If you've been unsuccessful in adding a better habit or ending an outdated habit, pay attention. Habits such as excessive sitting, overeating, drinking or smoking more than is aligned to your body goals, working too much, incessantly checking your devices, and staying up late are often effects of decision fatigue, which perpetuates itself by robbing tomorrow's energy to pay for today's endless activities. Over time, decision fatigue spirals downward, contributing to lack of focus and poor concentration, both of which lead to poor performance. Decision fatigue perpetuates both mental and physical stagnation, which compound epidemic levels of sedentary diseases borne of excessive sitting and inactivity. Inactivity increases the risk of cancers, anxiety, depression, heart disease, diabetes, and obesity. In fact, it now accounts for more deaths than smoking does.[9]

When you design your environments to prioritize smarter choices, your inner decision maker doesn't get fatigued. Here are some examples: First, say you want a more rejuvenating evening. Put a timer on your wireless router to power down after 9:00 p.m. You won't need to decide every night, when you're tired, about when to stop web-related activities, such as streaming or interacting with friends. Another example is the habit of eating dinner earlier to support going to bed earlier. A simple solution is to hang a big sign that says "Kitchen closed after 7:00 p.m.," reinforcing a desired habit through messaging. You might not have dinner wrapped up at 7:00 p.m. on day one, but now your environment is your habit reminder. Other ways to design your environment to reinforce the habits you want are setting out your clothes for the next morning's workout before you go to bed, cleaning your desk before you leave work for tomorrow's focused mind, putting cut vegetables in the doors of the fridge for easy access, switching to smaller plates for healthy portion sizes, and rearranging the garage or craft room to prioritize activities you enjoy. We'll explore more of this in the next chapter, on mastering earth, as you design habits to support your body's rhythms.

Perhaps you've noticed that when you wake up in the morning to a messy space with clothes and towels on the closet floor and mail and some dirty glasses on the kitchen counter, you feel stressed for the whole day. Perhaps you've noticed that when you start your morning with a clean closet and clean counters, you feel relaxed and in control for the day ahead. You can design your experience, that inner space of sthira, through a five- to ten-minute habit of putting everything away before you relax at night.

If you live with others, like I do, you might need to form a new group habit. Habits are formed by triggers. The five habit triggers are: a preceding action, a time, a place, another person, and an emotion.[10] The more triggers I involve, the easier I find it to build a group habit. After doing the dinner dishes (the preceding action trigger), I set a five-minute timer (the time trigger) for everyone (the other person trigger) to scour the house (the place trigger) to put the items they've used back in place and their personal items back in their own space. You could even play a certain song or two (the emotion trigger) when you start the timer. New habits have three parts: the trigger, then the new action, and then the reward. The trigger of the new habit is finishing the dishes, the new action is putting things in their places, and the reward is relaxation play time. Although it might take your family a week or two to build this practice into a habit, you'll enjoy each morning more. Any morning you wake up to a stress mess, you'll be invigorated to reinstate the habit. You are designing better habits *into your space*, reinforced by your enjoyment of your home.

Upholding sukha through intentionally freeing space of clutter involves many small habits. I focus on one-percent improvements in my home and office to set myself up for a better tomorrow. This generates ease and focus and a relaxed peak-performance environment. Small habits include putting stuff away immediately after use such as clothes and towels, keeping the sink and dish rack clear of dishes, and leaving my desk and office the way I want it to be when I arrive the next day.

Masters of space know that all is malleable, including our homes, habits, and personalities. Masters of space uphold an atmosphere of sukha (clean space, well-being), sthira (stillness, order, deep peace), and svastha (being seated in the self) to better intuit their dharma and receive that vision. They evolve their space ahead of the curve, meeting the next desires of dharma, enveloping their next mission in an atmosphere of thriving. As a result, their space triggers and supports the habits and inner atmosphere required for greater ease in their next mission. The inner rewards of sukha, sthira, and svastha root the master in the refined vibration of authenticity.

Congratulations, you're officially on the Master of You journey through the elements. You've synced your outer space to the emotional, mental, intuitive, and energetic atmosphere you want to have. In the next chapter, which focuses on earth element, you'll support your dharma through aligning your body rhythms for resilience and adaptability.

Use the following list to recognize your progress and inspire your next iteration of mastering space. Come back to this list time and again to measure your progress with space and point you forward.

MASTER OF SPACE (HOME)

○ You design your spaces based on the five
qualities you most want to experience.

○ Through sorting your stuff, you process emotions,
memories, past challenges, and even past identities.

○ Your ethos is reflected in your home, office, car, and storage
areas, reinforcing your own vibrant, creative vitality.

○ You build habits into your space to diminish
the effects of decision fatigue.

○ You take care of all your possessions knowing they
add value, meaning, and direction to your life.

○ Your spaces nurture your ambition, your body, and your spirit.

5

EARTH: MASTER OF BODY

N
ow that you designed your space to nurture your deeper
dreams into reality, it's time to turn to earth element to
gain the resilience to fuel your dharma, your ambitions.
From space to earth, we are moving from the subtlest element to the
most tangible, our roots. Mastering earth element means optimizing
our body rhythms to experience thriving. In this chapter, you will sync
your routines with your biological clock—your body's innate timing
device, which relies on day-and-night cycles—for daily nourishment,
more movement, and better sleep. This chapter is packed with simple
suggestions and quick tips. Remember, the aim is for a solid B– in your
experiments with mastering your body rhythms.

In Ayurveda, *prithvi*, or earth element, is the concept of all structure, form, solidity, and stability. Earth is the densest of the elements,
the most obvious to sense. Earth element in your body is the physical
matter, including the structure of your cells. The health of your cells,
tissues, and organ systems depends on aligning your habits to daily
and seasonal circadian rhythms. When you do, your cells pulse in harmony, detox, and regenerate. Aligned habits will extend your life and
help you feel rooted, independent, and vibrant throughout the cycles
of your life.

In yoga, this concept is known as root to rise. The deeper you root,
the higher you can extend. The rooting energy comes first in the equation seen in Figure 5.1.

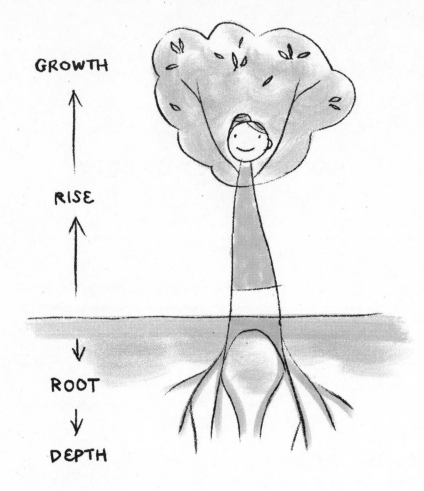

GROWTH

↑

RISE

↑

ROOT

↓

DEPTH

↓

Figure 5.1 Root to rise

This downward movement for upward pulsation is well understood by longevity practitioners. The more deeply you exhale, the more oxygen you can inhale. A complete morning bowel movement (downward energy) paves the way for healthier cravings (upward energy). Have you ever noticed this? The more deeply you consistently sleep, the more energy you have when you're awake. Or the hungrier you are, the more satisfying a good meal is. And have you noticed the opposite? If you eat when you're not very hungry, the meal isn't satisfying. When you don't sleep well, your mind and emotions aren't in great shape.

Aligned habits in waking and sleeping, hunger and satiation, workouts and recovery, a complete morning bowel movement for an empty colon, and peak performance and deep rejuvenation reorient you to thrive. According to Ayurveda, health is possible when the energy and intelligence within consciousness move in an effortless, pulsating flow through each cell. Strong pulsations set a rhythm. You are a being in action with a pulse, a beat, a rhythm—you are more of a verb than a noun. Your body is a living system that thrives on rhythm and falls apart when it's out of rhythm. From yoga, Taoism, and other ancient spiritual philosophies comes the concept that cosmic order generates daily and seasonal rhythms (called *rta* in Sanskrit and *Tao* in Taoism). Order gives rise to living in right relationship with purpose. When we are out of rhythm, we are at odds with dharma, or right action. Living out of sync with the cosmic order dis-integrates the connection between all five bodies. The experience is whole-body arrhythmia—irregularity with the beat of life. Modern science is onboard with this concept: "Irregular circadian rhythms have been linked to various chronic health conditions, such as sleep disorders, obesity, diabetes, depression, bipolar disorder, and seasonal affective disorder."[1]

Rhythm refers to a strong, synchronized, organic pattern. Etymologically, rhythm has roots in the word *flow*. When your basic body habits are aligned to the nighttime and daylight cycles, you have time and space on your side and feel in the flow of life. Health and resilience follow, opening the door to align your days to deeper meaning and higher purpose.

When your daily habits—eating, moving, sleeping—don't uphold your biological need for rhythm, your health suffers. Over time, you sacrifice mental clarity, focus, and peak performance—the key parts of the engine behind ambition. As a result, dis-ease can occur on the level of any of your five bodies (the five koshas, as explained in chapter 3): physically with chronic pain symptoms; emotionally with repetitive negative feelings; mentally with negative thought cycles about yourself and others; intuitively if you disconnect from your powers and lose presence, purpose, and spontaneity; and spiritually if your life loses deeper meaning.

Ayurveda has a saying, "Your body reflects your past," which points to how habits and experiences shape cells. Your cells are a snapshot of both past and present habits and experiences. They also indicate the trajectory of where your accumulated choices are leading next. Degenerative habits lead to cells functioning poorly and later malfunctioning. If your past habits are arrhythmic, you might have inflammation, hormone imbalances, skin issues, allergies, immune vulnerability, an accelerated heart rate or high pressure in your arteries and veins, shallow breathing, and loss of flexibility or strength.

The good news is that your body wants you to heed the cycles that build immunity, the bedrock of resilient longevity. In the words of Ayurvedic guru Robert Svoboda, "Your resilience, which is your capacity to roll with the punches and snap back to normal after even the lowest of blows, is your immunity."[2] You gain immunity by aligning your habits with the rhythms that support nourishment, movement, and sleep to fuel, detoxify, and rejuvenate. Daily habits also have a cumulative impact on your emotions, thoughts, energy level, healing, and resilience. Habits that support your body rhythms first heal you and then fuel your ambitions.

From an Ayurvedic perspective, understanding the koshas (the five bodies) and organizing your habits to fortify each body's unique intelligence lead to a healthy biological clock. However, when your habits make one body dominant, like a bully, you throw off your clock, sacrifice your health, and push dynamic harmony out of reach. For example, when your mind dominates, your attention is occupied with thinking versus movement or meditation. This is a factor in sedentary diseases, which I'll explore later.

Thankfully, to an impressive degree, aligning habits to our biological clocks and healthy circadian rhythms supports sleep, digestion, moods, and hormonal balance and turns around various chronic health conditions. As evidenced by research on epigenetics—the science of how diet and lifestyle habits influence genetic expression—humans can influence their own gene mutation as well as their muscle-to-fat ratio, body strength, and most other health indicators.[3] Use the Five-Bodies Check-in to determine the *think big, test small* experiments you might want to try to evolve your daily habits.

Five-Bodies Check-in

(You can listen to a recording of this exercise at masterofyou.us/
workbook.)

You now know that Ayurveda specifies five sheaths of the
self, the koshas, or five bodies. This exercise tunes you in to your
koshas so you can listen to and notice your body rhythms and
hear what needs your attention.

To access your koshas, start with deepening your breath.
Exhale. Inhale. Release. Expand your breath. Imagine that you
can slide your awareness from complexity to simplicity—to
unified rhythm. Next, check in with each body:

1. Bring your attention to your physical body.
   Be generally aware of any sensations. Is
   there any discomfort or pressure anywhere?
   Does your body feel heavy or light? Hot
   or cold? Inflamed? Relaxed or tense?

2. Now, direct your attention to your breath body.
   How do you feel as a breathing entity, as an energy
   body? Vibrant? Tired? Invigorated? Oxygenated?
   Or depleted? Is your breath shallow? Have your
   energy and moods swung high and low, or are they
   stable and reliable? Notice the breathing sensations,
   the pulsating of emptying and refilling. Do you
   feel anxious or calm? With practice, intentional
   breathing like this awakens and rejuvenates the
   breath body and calms the emotions and mind.

3. Next, shift your attention to your mind body—your
   emotions and thoughts. What emotions are you
   experiencing? What are the bodily sensations
   or breath patterns of those emotions or moods?
   Are the sensations dull or sharp? Hot or cold?
   Spreading or stuck? Pause to digest your

emotions through feeling the sensations. Then, become aware of your thoughts. Can you see a pattern in your thoughts from this week? Does that pattern lean toward positivity or negativity? Inclusiveness or isolation? Opportunity or overwhelm? Stress or ease? Frustration or just a change in perspective? Notice the physical sensations of that thought pattern. Pause to digest your thoughts through feeling the sensations.

4. Adjust your attention to your intuitive body. Ask your intuition, "What do I *want* to do tomorrow?" Don't listen to the *shoulds*. Listen for *wants* with your intuition. How does intuition communicate? Feel for sensations in your heart, your gut, your womb or lower belly, and your throat. Notice emotions. Notice thoughts. Notice your breath sensations as you feel for your wants.

5. Guide your attention to your spirit. Ask your spirit, "What do you want me to *hear* right now?" Listen for a moment. What messages does your spirit have for you? How do you hear the essence, the voice, the desires of your spirit? Linger in this conversation with your spirit for as long as it feels right.

With an attitude of self-compassion and curiosity, notice which of the bodies dominate and which are less accessible. Next, you'll assess your current habits and body rhythms and what you want in the next season of your life.

ENERGY AND MOVEMENT

Rate your satisfaction with your daily energy and movement on a scale of one to ten, where one is severely inadequate and ten is phenomenal. What is the quality or feeling of energy and amount of movement you want next?

SLEEP

Rate your degree of feeling refreshed on a scale of one to ten, where one is completely exhausted and ten is very well rested. What are your desires with regard to rejuvenation and sleep?

NOURISHMENT

Rate the degree of your body feeling nourished on a scale of one to ten, where one is not at all well nourished and ten is very well nourished. What would deep nourishment entail for you?

MOOD AND EMOTIONAL THRIVING

Rate your emotions on a scale of one to ten, where one is dismal and ten is delightful. Which specific emotions do you want to feel?

MUSCLE-TO-FAT RATIO

Rate your muscle-to-fat ratio on a scale of one to ten, where one is poor and ten is lithe and strong. How do you want your body to be and feel next?

Now you have intuitive data on your body rhythms. Pause to journal your desires and intentions. Reflection practices like this one are called *inquiry practices*, and they inform the path forward. Next, we'll treasure hunt for the easiest ways to find the gravitational pull into your body rhythms. ∎

THE THREE BODY RHYTHMS

From the Five-Bodies Check-in, you heard your body's desires for nourishment, movement, and rest. These are the three rhythms you want to fall into; when you have the rhythms dialed in, they become second nature. Like the force of gravity, these rhythms pull you into dynamic balance:

1. Rhythmic eating

2. Rhythmic movement

3. Rhythmic sleeping

As you read this chapter, you might generate reasons these body rhythms won't work for you, your lifestyle, or your body type. When that happens, remember your deeper dreams and return to your Five-Bodies Check-in notes, or do the practice again. This check-in moves your awareness into your cells and thereby into rhythm. Focus on small improvements—1 percent improvement per day—to orient yourself toward your vibrant longevity.

In chapter 3, we talked about the influence of culture on our thinking and our habits. Regarding the three body rhythms, modern culture is out of sync (see Figure 5.2). Simultaneously, many microcultures are positive influences that reinforce healthy body rhythms. Your microcultures include your family's culture, your friends' culture, your work environment, and those of the groups in which you're active. These all have their own ethos, beliefs, and accepted behaviors and exist in the larger culture of modern society. To more easily strengthen your body rhythms, attune to the microcultures around you with these healthier habits.

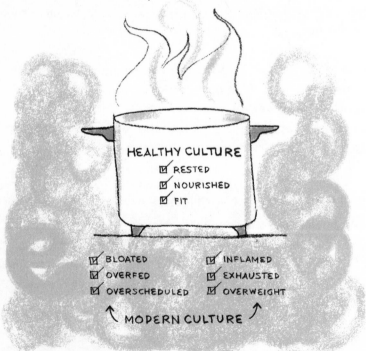

Figure 5.2 Cultures shape our habits, but healthy cultures can and do exist within unhealthy modern culture.

RHYTHMIC EATING: THE HUNGER AND SATIATION CYCLE

Bodies prefer rhythm, including in digestion and absorption. Unlike your heart and lungs, which are always working, your stomach and intestines need a long break. Many modern health problems stem from eating too frequently and not moving enough. Many people are eating *four to six times* a day, eating dinner late, and breaking their fast early. A simple reversal to eating no more than two to three times a day and physically moving often throughout the day solves many health problems.

Feeling good through the stages of life requires respect for feeding and fasting. Feeling emptiness turn into true hunger is an essential part of digestion upon which the pleasures of satiation depend. This involves feeling the *spanda*, or the pulsation of life—the full pulsation between the emptiness that arises when the stomach is empty and the fullness of digestion, when the prana, or life force, peaks. Many people rarely experience this, so it might take some getting used to before you come to welcome it. For multiple millennia, the yogis have applied rhythmic eating and fasting for spiritual clarity, natural daily cellular detox and renewal, and increased capacity both physically and mentally.

According to the Mayo Clinic, it takes about six to eight hours for a meal to move from your mouth and esophagus through your stomach and small intestines.[4] Similarly, Ayurveda advises adults to allow six hours between meals for optimal digestion. When you disrupt digestion by eating every few hours, overeating, eating too late, or eating when emotional, you incompletely digest your food. The by-product of incompletely digested food is called *ama*, or residue. Ama shows up first as symptoms ranging from bloating to constipation, excess stomach acid or diarrhea, or a heavy feeling in the stomach. If the root causes of ama aren't removed, it moves from the digestive tract through the bloodstream, affecting the mood with negative emotions. As it moves with the oxygenated blood to feed other cells, ama blocks the flow of the life force throughout the body. Ama is the opposite of conscious vitality. When digestion isn't completed, ama contributes to repressed emotions and eventually to mental confusion. It can move into organ systems, eventually isolating cells by coating the cell membranes and disrupting intercellular communication. This loss of intelligence weakens the immune response and can cause serious diseases such as autoimmune syndromes and cancer.[5]

You know you have ama if you wake up groggy, grumpy, stiff, bloated, or with bad breath. Bad breath is a strong indicator of chronic incomplete bowel movements or an unhealthy gut microbiome. When you eat rhythmically, your body develops a deeper efficiency with absorption and elimination. A healthy microbiome—with good gut bacteria—can replenish and thrive. You slow your body's aging by delegating energy for digestion and detoxification rather than mitigation of harmful habits.

Consider your eating rhythm last week. When did you eat? How much? How much time did you leave between meals and snacks? Your goal is a rhythm of nourishing and fasting so that you experience ease, energy, and mental focus. A fourteen- to sixteen-hour fasting time and eight- to ten-hour nourishment time is ideal for most people. In the process, you metabolize nutrients efficiently and shrink your stomach (losing excess belly fat) because your body more efficiently generates energy and healthy tissue.

Flip Your Fat

When you eat too frequently, the body doesn't use the calories stored in adipose (fat) tissue. When you space meals at least four to six hours apart, the adipose tissue burns slowly into stable energy, generating the relaxation response, which stabilizes mood and mind. Fat is a fuel source only when meals are spaced long enough apart for the blood sugar to drop, activating stored fat to be transitioned into energy. Fasting, or rhythmic meal spacing, also benefits your whole body because activated adipose tissue lubricates the joints and skin, creates cellular flexibility, generates a calm nervous system, and enhances intra- and intercellular communication. Snacking or eating too frequently spikes the blood sugar, and the fat gets locked out of circulation and stuck in storage.[6]

Ayurvedic and yogic research on meal spacing and fat metabolism, coupled with recent research from biohackers and longevity scientists, confirms that grazing throughout the day, overeating, or not allowing a long enough time between dinner and breakfast actually *disrupts* your body's natural rest-and-digest mode of fat metabolism.[7] This degenerative pattern of eating is part of the stress cycle.

Notably, fasting between meals strengthens your *agni*, or digestive fire, decreasing sensitivity to certain foods and generating a healthy appetite. However, snacking as a habit trains the body to source energy from the calories circulating in the blood. When you replenish your blood sugar every few hours with snacking, your body doesn't burn adipose tissue for fuel. Snackers train their bodies to crave food every few hours, which decreases their control over their appetites and leads to weight gain.[8] For snackers and frequent eaters, the drop in blood sugar after a few hours triggers their habit of eating rather than taking a digestive break that fuels the body from adipose tissue. Eating too frequently and overeating lead to excess adipose tissue, which becomes a place for excess calories that can't reenter circulation because of too frequent eating, creating a negative feedback loop tied to obesity and type 2 diabetes.[9] Also, the body moves toxins out of harm's way—to a storage site rather than into the organ systems—and chooses fat cells for this purpose. Toxins, including ama, are a result of repetitive and degenerative lifestyle choices. Skin issues, excess adipose tissue (such as belly fat), and joint pain are signs of unhealthy adipose tissue.

When people stop snacking and shift to less frequent meals, a transition occurs. During the transition they might have cravings, headaches, and unstable emotions. Yet, as their bodies rediscover adipose tissue as a fuel source, they recover appetite control, mood stability, and increased mental focus and experience fewer cravings, greater satiation, and better sleep. This is true for people with high and low blood sugar and diabetes. If you have issues with insulin or a type 2 diabetes diagnosis, consult a doctor or health practitioner that works with meal spacing.

Later in this chapter, I'll guide you through a one-week experiment; it takes about a week when switching from snacking to meal spacing for the body to rediscover the fuel stored in adipose tissue. After it does, cravings between meals subside, blood sugar stabilizes, and the mind becomes calm and focused. As your fat cells convert into energy, your body becomes leaner and detoxified, and you desire high-quality, nutrient-dense meals.

Emotional eating falls away when you take the time to feel your emotions. Processing the emotion rather than eating will shift your body from fight-or-flight mode into rest-and-digest mode. The next exercise, the WHO Breath, is helpful in disrupting the habit of snacking or emotional eating between meals. (The Five-Bodies Check-in is also a good one to try when stress arises.) This exercise helps you feel the movement in your digestive track. Remember spanda: first we want the downward, rooting energy, called *apana*. Then the upward rising energy, prana, follows.

The WHO Breath

(Listen to the recording of this exercise at masterofyou.us/workbook.)

Use the WHO breath to help curb the desire to eat between meals. This slow, deep, visceral breathing calms the mind and nerves, helps process emotions, and oxygenates the blood. The alimentary canal, or gastrointestinal tract, has a primitive simplicity, like that of an earthworm, as nutrients slide through phases of absorption. This practice can help you be more in touch with the fullness or emptiness in your stomach or intestines—and be able to make body-based decisions on whether you truly want more food in your body. Try a few WHO breaths when you want to eat but maybe shouldn't.

1. Inhale through your nostrils. Go slow.

2. Purse your lips together as if there is a straw between them.

3. Exhale, blowing through your imaginary straw. Slow and steady wins the race.

4. Listen for the sound WHO on the exhale.

5. Repeat ten times. You can use your fingers on your lap to count.

6. As you exhale, notice the muscles of your lungs, abdomen, and lower back. Notice what a complete exhale feels like. Notice the space you created for the next inhale. Notice what it feels like to be full and empty with breath.

7. Let your breathing return to normal while you sit, and notice the effects. Do you feel more content? Are you more in touch with your body's basic needs?

I learned this practice from modern yoga guru Donna Farhi, who teaches it to awaken awareness of digestive viscera. Some sections of your alimentary canal might feel open and free, whereas others feel stuck or dull. To reawaken those less spirited regions, try this practice every day for a month. ■

Introductory One-Week Experiment

With a one-week experiment in rhythmic eating, you can jump-start your fat metabolism and feel leaner, more energetic, and focused. You might also notice a decrease in symptoms of chronic inflammation (such as body pain, especially in the joints), poor digestion, low energy, skin rashes, and excessive mucus.[10] Start with a small experiment tomorrow: Have only water between meals. Think big and test small. Decide what times your meals will be, and aim for that rhythm. Carry a thermos to sip hot water between meals every twenty minutes to help with cravings. The hot water dissolves the ama and can alleviate headaches, body aches, or loose stools, which could happen if this process is detoxifying for you. Be self-compassionate by taking baths, going for walks, and doing self-massage.

After a few days of only water between meals, notice the fasting time between dinner and breakfast. Aim for a fourteen-hour fasting time overnight. In intermittent fasting, this is called a fourteen/ten, or a fourteen-hour fast and ten hours in which to eat.

If you fail fast, notice what got you off track. Then, shape the space in your kitchen or your schedule to help you adopt this habit. Aim for a little better. Don't rush this phase—you might naturally drift into the Moderate One-Week Experiment (below).

As you regain the sensations of emptiness and satiation, you'll recover the instinct to sense what nourishes you. "What should I eat?" is the number one question people ask holistic practitioners. With rhythmic eating, your cells will indicate what your body needs through healthy cravings. Trust your desires for vibrant, nutrient-dense food and lovely meals.

Moderate One-Week Experiment

As the Introductory One-Week Experiment begins working for you, your energy stabilizes, your stomach (belly fat) shrinks, and you'll be satisfied with more space between meals. The next phase is to gradually increase your nighttime fasting to fifteen hours, aiming for a fasting period from 6:00 p.m. to 9:00 a.m. to optimize digestion during daylight hours. Experiment with two to three meals a day, breaking your fast with a lighter meal—such as a green or red fruit-and-vegetable smoothie. Have a hearty lunch. For dinner, eat a less hearty meal. As a fifteen-hour nighttime fast becomes more comfortable, you can try a sixteen-hour fast, or a sixteen/eight fasting and eating schedule.

Tips for Rhythmic Eating

Use the Buddy System
Recruit a buddy to do this experiment with, and both of you aim for a solid B–! It's easier to evolve habits together.

Change *When* Before *What*
As you start with only water between meals and slowly extend the time between dinner and breakfast, don't focus on any other big changes in what you are eating.

→

Find Fabulous Fats

Your body will crave fabulous fats. Try avocado, tahini, coconuts, and soaked almonds and cashews. Make dressings and sauces with high-quality, organic, cold-pressed oils, such as olive, avocado, or walnut. If you are an omnivore, buy organic whole birds, such as chickens or turkeys, and use the skin and bones for bone broth. The fat in the skin and the marrow is deeply soothing to the nerves and decreases emotional food cravings for sweets, pastries, and artificial foods.

Focus on Fun Time

You'll have more time in your life from less-frequent meal preparation and cleanup, less waiting in restaurants, and not dealing with the chronic health issues. Focus on activities you love in the evening and early morning, such as walking, reading, visiting, playing with your kids, yoga, gardening, and meditating.

Break Your Fast with Phytonutrients

Break your fast each morning with phytonutrient-rich fruits and juices made from veggies, fruits, and water. Phytonutrients are natural plant chemicals that enhance immunity and intercellular communication, repair DNA damage from exposure to toxins, detoxify carcinogens (lowering your risk of cancer), and reduce inflammation and the risk of heart disease.[11] For example, make a purple smoothie that enhances digestion and elimination with an apple, ½ of a small beet, a handful of blueberries, a few stalks of celery, purple kale, a cup of water, and a cup of pomegranate juice. Notice the life force in these living foods and enjoy the buzz of natural energy they give you.

Love Your Body with Self-Massage

Self-massage aids in detoxification and transformation of adipose tissue. In the evening, give yourself a massage with quality, organic, cold-pressed oils, such as sesame, coconut, or avocado. For an even more decadent experience, mix in a few drops of essential oil, such as lavender or chamomile. You'll sleep better too!

→

Traveling and Socializing

If you eat later with others, focus on your hearty lunch. When traveling, you might find it socially convenient to switch to having dinner by 7:00 p.m., a green drink in the late morning, and a meal between 11:00 a.m. and 1:00 p.m. When you're done traveling, readjust to eating earlier. If you eat alone, you might gravitate toward an 8:00 a.m. to 4:00 p.m. feeding interval.

Two "Real" Meals

Switching from three meals a day to two meals most days simplifies life, generates time, and can stabilize your energy for prolonged mental clarity and physical strength. Food sensitivities to many modern exiled foods, including grains, legumes, gluten, and dairy, might also disappear as your digestion becomes robust. Pack your first meal of the day with nutrient-dense proteins and fats, such as an avocado, eggs with swiss cheese, sourdough toast, and steamed greens with butter to fortify you for six hours. Make your evening meal hearty enough to last until the next day.

RHYTHMIC MOVEMENT

As your physiology becomes more efficient and easeful from rhythmic eating, your instinct to move more takes over. As bipedal primates, we evolved to standing and walking, freeing our hands for tools.

Yet, the desk job and couch potato mode are disastrous, degenerative, contemporary fads gone global and viral. The effects of the global rise in "sedentary diseases" are alarming. People who sit still for more than four hours per day have a 40 percent higher disease risk than those who sit fewer than four hours per day.[12] Less than 20 percent of Americans have physically active jobs.[13] The higher health risks of a sedentary lifestyle include obesity, heart disease, high blood pressure, high cholesterol, stroke, type 2 diabetes, cancer, migraines, and so forth.[14] Adopting active lifestyles could reduce all types of cancer rates by as much as 46 percent.[15] These numbers are staggering.

There is clear evidence of an inverse relationship between volume of physical activity and mortality rates in men, women, younger adults, and older adults. With only minimal physical activity, people lose 20 to 30 percent of their life span. The more diverse the physical activity that dominates your daily life—not necessarily "working out"—the further you reduce your health risks.[16]

Lack of frequent physical activity—or rhythmic movement—is also a recipe for emotional disaster. After surveying more than 3,300 government employees, Australian researchers found that men who sat for more than six hours a day at work were 90 percent more likely to feel moderate psychological distress—such as feeling nervous, restless, hopeless, or tired—than men who sat for less than three hours a day.[17] Modern sedentary culture has overridden the natural instinctual desire to get up and walk, stretch, or be active multiple times a day.

Yet, modern culture even emphasizes a way of exercising that isn't rhythmic but rather based on a once-a-day or every-other-day "workout." "Working out" implies labor, which for many inactive people is unappealing, strenuous drudgery. Modern "workouts" trade in a natural diversity of movement for one type of "exercise" per day, such as jogging, calisthenics, or lifting weights, and often focus on calorie burning or strengthening specific muscle groups to achieve a certain look.

What we actually need is to move more frequently and functionally throughout the day. Functional movement is exploratory exercise that enhances how you move all day. It's a mix of crawling, walking, squatting, reaching, lunging, jumping, rolling around, rocking, and moving from the floor to standing to back to the floor. In modern culture, functional movement often ends with childhood, so watch the movements of toddlers and kids at play. They choose movement out of a desire to explore, with no conscious concern for strengthening their muscles or burning off their previous meal. They often move their four limbs in multiple planes: forward, backward, sideways, and on and off the floor, which enhances coordination and aggregates strength. All of that stems from rolling, crawling, lunging, and climbing. This unpremeditated and unpredictable movement for the toddler is functional—a means to an end. Functional movement for adults sparks better biomechanics for doing everyday actions such as picking up a sock off the floor, reaching overhead to remove luggage from the airplane bin, getting up and down from the floor without using hands, or squatting to rest without needing a chair. Classes for functional movement and natural movement are searchable on YouTube and popping up in gyms.

Rhythmic movement means adding a variety of natural physical activities frequently throughout your day. Frequency wins over intensity as you slowly recover your body's natural instinct to move. If you don't move every hour or two, you sacrifice your ability to focus and remain refreshed throughout the day. Although you might exercise daily, you also want to find opportunities to move frequently throughout the day. A typical day with rhythmic movement might include beginning the day with five to twenty minutes of stretching or exercise, taking "movement breaks" throughout the day, getting in your 10,000 steps by walking more frequently, jumping on the trampoline with the kid after school, *and* bicycling around the neighborhood after dinner. Just as when a two-year-old wakes up or finishes eating, pivot into a few minutes of movement if you've been sedentary for more than an hour during the day. If frequent movement is not yet a habit for you, give yourself a break—our culture encourages a mostly sedentary lifestyle beginning with our first day at school. In conventional classrooms, children are indoctrinated into unnatural, disease-causing, sedentary, physical sedation, talked *out* of natural functional movement, and often medicated with pharmaceuticals if they don't acquiesce.

Add more movement here and there throughout your day with physical work, play, and any other type of movement that gets your heart and lungs pumping. Arouse your intrinsic desire to move! At home, take breaks from screen time by doing housework, gardening, taking social walks and bike rides, and exercising. Ten minutes of vacuuming, carting laundry around (not sitting and folding), a quick break to organize the garage, and pulling some weeds all count. You will discover a new set point—a new normal that you know guarantees a vibrant day.

Eventually, you'll find all sorts of movement becoming part of your normal day, every day, even when traveling or when visitors or crises throw off your routines. In the beginning, you might have to drag your body up from the chair, so start small: try a walk around the building or a few jumping jacks.

Rhythmic Movement at Work and Home

Begin your day with five to twenty minutes of breath-body movement to establish the breath and access your intuition, spirit, positive emotions, and inspired thinking for the day ahead. Then, to recover the joy and health benefits of rhythmic movement, note a few ideas from the lists below and try them this week.

HOME IDEAS

- Start your day with a functional movement video on YouTube (I like the channel Movement Parallels Life).

- Do housework in spurts, wear ankle weights, put on a headset, and dance while you vacuum or do laundry.

- Garden and landscape in short stints.

- Walk to your neighbor's house, or go for a walk with your neighbor.

- Ride your bike to the store.

- Walk around the park and throw in CrossFit exercises while the kids play.

- Do a few jumping jacks or side stretches.

- Stand or walk when you are talking on the phone.

- Stretch while watching TV.

WORK IDEAS

- Take the stairs.

- Use a wireless headset, and pace when you are talking on the phone.

- Use a standing or treadmill desk.

- Have a walking or standing meeting.

- Walk to someone's desk rather than sending an email.

- Walk or bike to work.

- Stretch for one minute after you use the bathroom.

RHYTHMIC SLEEP

At last, we turn to sleep: *early to bed, early to rise makes a human healthy, wealthy, and wise.*

The earth spinning on its axis, generating night and day, shapes the rhythms of life forms on this planet. Rhythmic sleeping happens when you follow the downward pull of the setting sun, reliably sleeping eight hours, ideally from around 9:00 p.m. to 5:00 a.m. Your ambition requires you to show up consistently well rested. When you align with this circadian rhythm, rejuvenation happens. When you don't, you risk chronic disease from disrupting your body's endocrine intelligence.

Sleep duration in the general human population has decreased by one and a half to two hours per night, around 25 percent, from nine hours to less than seven, since the early 1900s.[18] As a global culture, we are no longer sleeping rhythmically, which has led to massive erosion of immune function in modern humans and widescale chronic disease. The US Centers for Disease Control (CDC) reports that one-third of adults report habitually getting less than the recommended amount of sleep. The CDC also reports that chronically shortchanging sleep leads to many diseases and conditions such as type 2 diabetes, heart disease, obesity, and depression, not to mention increased likelihood of accidents and injuries. Even six to seven hours of sleep per night slowly increases inflammation levels and destroys immune function.[19]

The effects of sleep deprivation and arrhythmic rest are slow to accumulate. Sleep-deficient individuals often perceive that they are operating normally, which makes it hard to catch and reverse or avoid devastating side effects. Of fatal accidents in the United States, 20 percent involve a drowsy driver.[20] Memory issues, coupled with poor concentration and decreased problem-solving ability, result in sleep-deprived people underprepared to reverse the situation. Most don't realize their insufficient sleep is driving their excess caloric intake, drawing them into an endless negative emotional loop, diminishing their sex drive, increasing their accident-proneness, causing chronic inflammation and poor immunity, and reducing their ability to solve the problem of their sleep deprivation.

If you don't wind down with the sun, you train your body to produce cortisol around 8:00 p.m.[21] This stimulating hormone is a key player in the chronic endocrine disruption pattern, raising stress hormones, such as insulin; reducing leptin, which helps you feel full; and raising ghrelin, an appetite stimulant, which leads to weight gain.[22] For many, this wired-and-tired cycle leads to obesity and poorer performance of all activities. As your stress hormones such as cortisol increase, your sex hormones, such as oxytocin, estrogen, and progesterone decrease, affecting healthy libido, pleasure, and fertility.[23]

The good news is that with rhythmic eating and movement, you set yourself up for rhythmic sleeping. The more you want to experience or accomplish in your life, the more incentive you have to deepen your sleep with a relaxing evening ritual.

Ritualize Rhythmic Rest

By the end of the day, you have accumulated experiences, emotions, thoughts, and ideas. Rhythmic rest involves creating an iterative ritual that declutters your mind and relaxes your body, incrementally lengthening and improving your sleep. A ritual is an act regularly repeated in a precise manner according to a set sequence, usually performed in a sequestered place. Aim to back up your current bedtime to 9:30 or 10:00 p.m. in fifteen-minute increments per night. Write down your sequential rest ritual to test this week, and tape it to your bathroom mirror or fridge. Weekly, rewrite your ritual to refine what is working.

IDEAS FOR BUILDING A REST RITUAL

- Put your phone/tablet/computer to bed at a certain time each evening.

- Set out exercise clothes for the next morning.

- Stretch or do yoga.

- Meditate.

- Give yourself a foot massage.

- Journal for a few minutes.

- Turn out the lights by 9:30 or 10:00 p.m.

Adopt a *kaizen* mindset, which means striving for doable, incremental, but continuous improvement.

Master Your Constitution: Learn Your Dosha

To prioritize a body rhythm on which to focus first, look through the lens of your constitution. Vata types become anxious or overwhelmed without daily regularity in meals and sleep, which becomes the bedrock to thriving in relationships, health, and dharma. Pitta types

→

should focus on their bedtime routine and movement breaks as well as local and seasonal nutrient-dense, organic foods for peak rejuvenation. Kapha types thrive when they emphasize sixteen- to eighteen-hour fasting times and an early morning movement habit.

ABX: ALWAYS BE EXPERIMENTING

Everything you do is an experiment that gives instantaneous feedback. To align your body rhythms, remember the code: "Think big, test small, fail fast, learn always." Activate your rhythms with 1 percent improvement per day. This will result in new experiences and new perspectives. Your dreams always think big, so partner with your potential by looking to your five bodies to decide which small, meaningful experiments to do. Be willing to fail and learn.

Master your body rhythms for the resilience to power your ambition. Run on a full tank of energy, and continually replenish yourself to experience more ease, more resilience, and more capability. To master earth element is to root and reroot rhythms in your cells. Your body thrives on ritualistic routines revolving around rhythm. Fall into this ancient circadian flow to rebalance your endocrine system.

Remember, you are wired for bliss at any age. Your body craves rhythm and attention. You are on a journey into deeper cellular embodiment. Cooperate with your physiology through rhythmic nourishment, movement, and sleep, and your body will unveil the delights of subtle ease, bliss, and interconnectivity. This positive feedback loop will reveal itself when you fall into rhythm. The more interconnected your cells, the better you will feel, the more positive emotions you will experience, the more interconnected you can become in your relationships, and the more intuitively easeful you will become in your decision making. You will become increasingly integrated from spirit through body, from idea through prototype. Get curious about who you can become next. How resilient can you be so that you can lead a life with a bigger purpose?

MASTER OF EARTH (BODY)

◯ You eat in rhythm, conscious of fasting times.

◯ Your bones carry the right amount of muscle and fat.

◯ You run on fat metabolism in rest-and-digest mode.

◯ You expand your daily repertoire of functional movement.

◯ You begin every day with movement or a workout.

◯ You break up your day with physical activities.

◯ You ritualize your rest to go to bed before 10:00 p.m. and consistently get eight hours of good sleep for rejuvenation.

◯ You kaizen body experiments to build your resilience.

◯ You fuel your ambition from the circadian rhythms.

6

FIRE: MASTER OF AMBITION

As your living and working spaces and body rhythms align with your purpose, your ambition comes into focus, revealing your dharma. Dharma reveals itself through your specific desires, an emerging vision of what you want your life to be like next. In space element, we focused on your home and workplace, in earth element we addressed your body rhythms, and in fire element we now turn to the powers of your mind. Fire element in the Master of You system focuses on mental powers, the capacity to discern your vision and forge your best strategy into a plan of action.

In this chapter, you'll begin by shining the light on your past. You'll write your personal history to get a clear sense of who you've been. Your history is the fuel for who you are becoming and generates the light to clearly see your next unique opportunities and challenges. Then, you'll go on a quest for your three-year vision. Focusing your mental fire, you'll determine a strategy—your best route forward—that accounts for potential issues as best as you can forecast them.

Take note: this chapter includes exercises easier *to read* than they are *to do*! Moving ambition forward into reality is profound and challenging work that pays off in your next months, years, and decades. By engaging in the exercises and learning this process over time, you develop a better, and often unexpected, strategy to move your dreams into reality.

A BURNING DESIRE TO ALIGN
YOUR ACTIONS: *TAPAS*

Tejas, or fire, is the most intense and transformative of the five elements. Fire requires the spark of desire, fuel for sustenance, and space to spread. In the Master of You system, we apply fire's sharp mental energy to decipher the best plan of action in getting there. According to Ayurveda, the qualities of fire element are hot, intense or sharp, clear, and forward moving. You can direct the light of fire to help you decide your destination. With the power of discernment fire brings, you burn off all other options. You process the lessons you've learned in your life, and as a result, you discover your best assets and opportunities for the journey ahead in order to create a strategy and then a plan.

Yogis historically have held a special regard for fire element. The term *tapas*, or intentional friction, is regarded as key to enlightenment, to transforming the mundane into the extraordinary. Tapas is generated from the tension of taking necessary, informed actions to evolve—similar to the experience of a tough, sweat-inducing workout. Tapas transforms what already is into the fuel for what is possible next. In burning off other possibilities, you decide your best route forward. Tapas also purifies and directs your next identity by burning off what no longer serves you, generating light to reveal the way forward. Seeing right effort and aligned effort, versus more effort, is fire's gift of self-compassion and self-realization.

The exercises to master fire element activate tapas by raising your bar, aligning your actions, and requiring you to own your results. You'll begin where you are—in the busyness of modern life, which absorbs free time like a sponge. Your goal is to get out of the weeds, climb the metaphorical mountain, and gain a viewpoint. With the direction of fire to align your actions, you will rise like a phoenix out of the ashes. Give yourself the time to do the exercises in this chapter, beginning with writing your story.

YOUR STORY IS THE FUEL FOR YOUR FIRE

Your history is the fuel for your future. You want a clear picture of who you have become, where you are standing now, in order to recognize specifically and articulately what you bring to the table of your future.

Clinical psychologist and Harvard professor Jordan B. Peterson writes in *12 Rules of Life*, "You must determine where you have been in your life so you can know where you are now. If you don't know where you are precisely, then you could be just about anywhere." Not one to mince words, Peterson continues, "You must determine where you have been in your life, because otherwise you can't get to where you're going."[1] To do this, you start by discovering key strengths, unforgettable lessons, and the critical situations that forged you. Peterson further explains, "As you own your story, you plant your flag in the Earth. You are here now. You will better know and own who you've been, who you are, and who you are becoming."[2]

There is a story to who you have become. By collecting the threads of your past, you illuminate, articulate, affirm, and update who you are now. In remembering, and bringing the parts of you together, you weave the threads of your past into the fabric of who you are now.

Write Your Story

(You can also listen to a guided audio recording and find a worksheet for this exercise at masterofyou.us/workbook.)

Choose how you will capture the threads of your story, such as journaling, drawing a story board, sketching a time line, or speaking your story into a recording or transcription app.

By answering the following questions, you'll be better able to formulate the best strategies, which lead to your deeper dreams. You want to capture your tools, traumas, breakthroughs, and patterns in your story. If you have a hard time looking back, focus on the positive, celebrating your uniqueness and what makes your story yours and the challenges you have overcome.

1. Think back to what mattered most to you as a child. What brought you the most joy?

2. Recall your highs and lows as a teen and young adult—your breakdowns and breakthroughs.

3. What big breakthroughs have you had in your adult life? Consider your health, relationships, family, career, money, service to others, and even your personality.

4. What do you uncompromisingly stand for as a result of your experience?

5. Who most helped you become what you are most proud of?

6. What parts of your past, phases, or patterns now feel complete?

7. What stage are you entering now? How does it feel? In what qualities of yourself do you now feel rooted?

That's it. For Master of You purposes, you just wrote your story thus far. Take a moment to honor yourself for pausing to weave the web of who you have become and for being willing to do the work. In this process, you absorb own your wisdom, strengths, lessons learned, and weaknesses to inform the strategy for your heroine's journey ahead. You are ready to go on a quest for your three-year vision. ∎

Master Your Constitution: Learn Your Dosha

When approaching your ambitions with vision, strategy, and planning, it can help to keep your dosha, or constitution, in mind. If your mental constitution is pitta—meaning you are mentally sharp and naturally logical and discerning—you might find yourself fully engaged, a natural, in the arena of vision-planning. If your mental constitution is vata—meaning you are naturally enthusiastic and have high, quick-start energy—use those strengths to plow through the exercises, not overthinking them. Let loose your creativity and morph

→

the exercises to suit your personality. If your mental constitution is kapha, don't procrastinate on generating a strategy; remember that it will save you effort down the road. Do the exercises first thing in the morning. Find a buddy if that helps. For all types, remember these exercises are designed to guide you into actions you wouldn't otherwise take that lead you to an even better life.

QUEST FOR YOUR THREE-YEAR VISION

When Justicia started with the Master of You group, she didn't have a clear vision of her future. She couldn't sense her next dharma. A business partner to her husband and a yoga teacher, her kids all grown, she was going through the motions of life without any spark. In the process of writing her story, she was struck by her past success as a painter. This part of her was swept under the rug for more than twenty years. From engaging in the exercises around dreaming, mining regrets and yearnings, aligning to her body rhythms, and writing her story, she was ignited to paint. She picked up painting again and was overcome with the shakti of it, the power. Her spark was back. She invited her husband to do the Master of You exercises with her, including developing their three-year vision together. Their vision included her exiting the company, the two of them finding a perfect fit for a new business partner, her painting and showing her work in galleries and earning a premium, having a helper take care of aging parents, and buying a second home—a cabin in the woods in Germany. Astonishingly, within eight months, they had achieved their three-year vision. This is the power of gaining mastery with the elements.

Although these results are astounding, I've found that achieving smaller dreams brings the same amazing feeling. For instance, Amy became pregnant after years of trying. After she had her baby, she continued to work and rework the five-element process of Master of You. A talented organizer, she realized around six months postpartum that she wanted to work only a few hours a week. By honoring her story and her deeper dreams, she was able to arrange her life to be a full-time mom. She is happier than ever.

Now is the time to *think big*. Rooted in your story, you are prepared to pursue your three-year vision. Three years is the sweet spot between the infinite future and now; it's a mini forever, a trilogy of iterations possible within a decade. This solid chunk of time is malleable enough for the mind to manage, yet long enough for a lot to happen.

When you consider three years out, you set yourself up for something great. The term a *big hairy audacious goal* (BHAG) captures the spirit of you doing something great.[3] Yet, this can also spin some people into perpetual stress; they might be better off considering a goal that simply feels aligned, smart, resilient, and grounded. Trust your desire in knowing how big or small you want to be next. For some, a BHAG might be reducing 50 percent of your work for time to travel and play. Paul Jarvis, author of *Company of One: Why Staying Small Is the Next Big Thing for Business*, reminds people who want to enjoy their lives that they can also set goals that focus specifically on the life they want, which might be smaller, smarter, more efficient, and more resilient.[4]

You'll start your quest with the question, "What exactly am I aiming for in the next three years?" Author and Jungian analyst Clarissa Pinkola Estés points out, "Asking the proper questions is the central action of transformation. Questions are the key that causes the secret doors of the psyche to swing open."[5] What do you want more of in your life? What do you want less of in your days? Recall the five words you generated when you mastered your space, and recall your superheroine image. Your three-year vision should feel good, exciting yet grounded, and svastha—seated in your uniquely personal self. With aligned effort, it should feel possible or at least plausible. To receive your vision, I recommend you go on a short quest, a pilgrimage of sorts. Examples abound of people going on a mission, a quest, a pilgrimage to see beyond what they can normally see. Our myths across time and cultures describe the process of leaving the herd, stepping outside the status quo to see a brighter future. Seekers are willing to trade their past stories of themselves for future possibilities. The pioneer trades in chatter for silence, the known for the unknown, the predictable for the incalculable, engaging tapas in the process.

To bring your three-year vision to front and center, schedule time for a quest soon. This time investment up front compounds like interest, saving you headaches and delays in the future by aligning your actions now.

Quest for Your Three-Year Vision

If you're able, schedule a half or full day for your vision quest. You are doing a ritual to cross the threshold from your ordinary thinking into possibility thinking. I recommend getting out of your normal schedule or habitual environment to think outside your box. Liminal thinking—thinking beyond the threshold of your regular or conditioned mind—will open up your vision quest.[6] Plan your day to sit to capture thoughts, walk to process ideas, and eat good food, perhaps going to a public library, favorite cafe, and local park with a pad of paper or a laptop. Or you might hike to a special spot with your journal or stay home to use poster-sized sticky notes on the walls.

Note: if you are doing this in a group—with coworkers or family—follow the same order as I describe below, giving time for both personal reflection and group discussion (for the prompts, change the "I" to "We").

1. Prepare (ten minutes): Plan where you'll go and what you'll need, including a journal and colorful pens to map your vision. Plan a schedule that includes time for walking and stopping to do the steps below. As you prepare, ask yourself, "What exactly am I aiming for in the next three years?" You can repeat the question to yourself, emphasizing the different words: *what, exactly, I, aiming, three.*

2. Start (ten minutes): Start your quest with a small ritual such as lighting a candle, smudging the space around you with a sage stick, or

meditating for one minute, to clarify your intention and move your awareness into liminal thinking. Today is for thinking big. What exactly are you aiming for in the next three years?

3. Contemplate and ideate (two hours): Consider what you want to be like in three years. What do you want your life to be like? What do you want your body to feel like? Who is the person you dream of becoming? Are you being called to some purpose? What is that, exactly? What do you want to be doing with your time three years from now? With whom? This day is meant for you to ask the big questions. Record what you are thinking, feeling, and desiring. Draw pictures or stick figures. Capture your words, circle, and highlight. Recall your superheroine from chapter 3.

4. Take movement and nourishment breaks (one to two hours): Break up your day by asking these questions during a walking contemplation exercise. Eat a good meal. Pay attention to what you are noticing; you might see symbols around you that clarify your vision. Drink plenty of water to keep your mind alert. Remember, this is your day to think big.

5. Record (two hours): Review your notes from the day so far. Return to the questions, letting your thoughts circulate. Draw a picture of your three-year vision. Add words. Clarify what you want in your life and where your dharma is leading. Trust your desires. If you feel stagnant or tired, take a moment to sit in silence, or if it is convenient, take a cold shower to refresh your mind. Looping an ambient song can help with deeper concentration. I prefer pianists such as Nils Frahm, Max Richter, and Joep Beving. Vision quests are intense work.

End with a clear picture and/or page of writing
that summarizes your three-year vision.

6. Wrap up your day with a three-year vision
   statement. Select the key, specific outcomes from
   your notes. Edit your words into one sentence:
   an accurate, specific, clear, succinct, trimmed
   statement expressing the specific outcomes
   you will achieve within the next three years.
   Check that your three-year vision resonates
   with all five bodies (you can do the Five-Bodies
   Check-in exercise from chapter 5 to confirm).

7. Celebrate with deep replenishment and deep
   rest. Congratulations on time well invested. With
   a lucid three-year vision, it's strategy time. ■

THE SLOW ROAD TO FASTER RESULTS

Lao Tzu wrote, "The slow overcomes the fast." In my twenties and thirties, I would set goals and take immediate actions. Through failing fast and spinning my wheels, I learned Lao Tzu's lesson. Rather than springing into action on your big vision, the exercises in this chapter are designed to help you slow down now to go faster later. Fire is sharp, and this sharpness of mind, this disciplined practice, is groundwork for a smoother journey later. As Abraham Lincoln reportedly advised, you are investing your time sharpening the axe before you chop down the tree.[7]

Unlike space, which expands; air, which can blow in any direction; or water, which meanders downstream, fire always creates heat that rises. These fire element exercises and practices awaken tejas, an intense inner power that illuminates and shines from within. Tejas arises out of right action, including aligned thinking. The exercises in this book are a krama, a specific sequence of steps that build upon each other. This heavy-thinking, up-front sequence stokes your mental faculties to generate a well-thought-out strategy you can rely on later. You will have transformed, lit up with tejas, in the process.

You've come through the work of unearthing your dreams, redesigning your home, building resilient body habits, writing your story, and conceiving your three-year vision. This is the starting place, your A. Your three-year vision actualized is the finish line, your B. Now you need a foolproof plan to get from A to B. The opportunity at hand is in the answers to the questions: *What will you need to make it happen? What will you need to do for your vision to become real? What could keep you from making this happen?* You are bringing to the surface your critical issues regarding this vision.

With a three-year vision, you will naturally have gaps in the skills, resources, assets, and relationships needed to get there. Gaps mean you are interested in developing yourself as a human being. Good thing you have plenty of time to build skills, resources, and assets and to develop relationships. Your job now is to gather the data that will help you map the best road to get there, by assessing what you have that will help you and what you don't have that you will need. In the next exercise, you'll bring to light your strengths and weaknesses, which will reveal your critical issues and the crucial opportunities to help you make your vision real.

SWOT

This exercise takes only an hour or so. The SWOT is a preliminary exercise used by businesspeople to gather data before building a solid strategy. If you've learned this at work but haven't applied it to your personal or family goals, carpe diem. I've used it for years to gather the data for a strategy to hit my personal goals, to help my team hit our company goals, and with my family for our lifestyle-design and wealth goals. Either alone or as a team, you will identify the strengths, weaknesses, opportunities, and threats circulating around your three-year vision. Later, these data will point to your critical issues to overcome.

To start this exercise, I recommend putting four big pieces of paper on a wall; or, if you don't have room, use four big pieces of paper at your table. I use poster-size sticky notes, but big pieces of paper taped to the wall work well for viewing your SWOT from a distance later. Label each paper with one category:

1. Strengths

2. Weaknesses

3. Opportunities

4. Threats

Next, read your three-year vision aloud. Sit with your *think big* vision. See your desired future as real. Then, spend fifteen minutes on each category to write down everything that *might be connected to achieving or falling short of your vision*. Set judgment aside; humility and honesty with yourself now will pay dividends later. I'll walk you through the four categories:

1. Strengths: In light of your three-year vision, you have specific strengths to leverage to get there. What are they? Be specific. Revisit your strengths and native genius from the assessments you did in chapter 3. Consider what others have said about you, including compliments you have received. Your strengths might have been generated through iterative practice. Include natural abilities, relationships, or assets that can help you achieve your vision. Strengths beget unique opportunities. Capture these aces in your sleeve so that you can use them to amplify your strategy. Rehash your biggest accomplishments, hard-won achievements, and tough lessons learned. They surfaced earlier in your story. What makes you capable of pursuing your three-year vision?

2. Weaknesses: Now, you want to excavate any weaknesses that could derail your three-year vision. Recall the breakdowns from your story exercise earlier in this chapter—to forecast recurring patterns that blindside you, slow you down, or hold back your progress. Set judgment aside in exchange for a clear assessment. Look for problems you wish you had already resolved; challenges that keep reappearing; or skills, assets, knowledge, or relationships you don't have that might be key to reaching your goal. These gaps, if you can find them earnestly, are gold nuggets for your strategy. There is nothing to fear—a good strategy will pair your critical weaknesses with assets, key relationships, and other strengths. Get them on the table.

3. Opportunities: Next, look for current situations or potential future circumstances that might be favorable to your three-year vision. What are they? What could easily advance your success with your vision? What is easy for you to grow or move forward fast in your vision? Some opportunities come from particular connections, others from the changing marketplace—locally, regionally, or globally. Still others come from unique abilities you've developed.

4. Threats: Last but not least, identify the risky unknowns of your three-year vision. What could stop you? What might be beyond your control? What situations or circumstances might arise that could undermine what you're trying to make happen? Pinpoint potential threats, even those less likely but still concerning, to inform your vision when it comes to building your strategies.

Now, circle the big guns in your data (the things that will most definitely help or hurt you).

With your SWOT well on its way, you might find it useful to keep your papers on the wall for a week. If you did this as a working group or family, keep them on the wall and add to them throughout the week. If you can, review your findings with someone outside the circle, an interested friend or colleague. They might point out strengths or a threat you overlooked or identify a certain opportunity you did not envision.

That is all you need to do for now. You have a very good data set for building your strategy. ■

ILLUMINATING YOUR CRITICAL ISSUES

As Brian Moran, author of the *The 12 Week Year*, reminds us, "A vision without a plan is a pipe dream."[8] The fire of the mind is required to blaze a path forward. When you consider your SWOT in light of an ambitious vision, issues might rise to the surface. *Critical issues* is a term used by business strategists to identify what needs to be tackled in order to make a smart action plan. (Yogis might call them *critical karmas* to highlight the path between cause and effect.) Critical issues surface mostly because of competing interests, limited resources, unknowns about opportunities, and threats bigger than they appear. Critical issues surface from answering the questions, "What could go wrong? What obstacles must you overcome?"

"Discrimination is the mind's digestion, which determines whether or not a course of action is appropriate for the well-being of the organism," states Ayurvedic doctor Robert Svoboda.[9] Discrimination, or discernment, Svoboda points out, is the mental equivalent of fire in Ayurveda and is required to find the best course of action out of the many possibilities.[10] This friction of focused thinking generates the glow of insight. A strategy generated from disciplined thinking allows aligned actions to fall into place. Strategy is formed from thorough processing of the critical issues. These processes of structured thinking focus attention like a laser on a deliberate future. Profound insights and spiritual breakthroughs are part of solid strategic planning.

Critical issues require narrowing all the potential problems and opportunities into what must receive attention in order for the vision to be possible. Critical issues chisel the three-year vision into a question: "What are my essential strategies to make this dream happen?" How should I get from A to B? Razor-sharp, fiery attention rather than Pollyannaish thinking is needed to find the route through the challenging terrain ahead.

Use these question stems to identify critical issues: "How might I . . . ?" or "How do I . . .?" For example, a family might generate this issue: *How might we live abroad for a year (three-year vision) given that we can't cover our home mortgage (weakness or strength) and rent a place abroad (opportunity)?* The strategy this question suggests is researching solutions such as renting out their home or perhaps trading houses. Strategic issues I've had in the past include, "How might I spend more time with my kid (opportunity tied to three-year vision) while writing a book and running a company (strength)?" J. P. Morgan says, "No problem can be solved until it can be reduced to some simple form."[11] Channeling the vision into the best plan is the strategic quest.

Business strategist Tyler Norton says that the best strategies arise from the intersections of certain strengths, weaknesses, opportunities, and threats to solve for the most critical issues to move your dreams forward.[12] Considering what could hold you back or propel you forward, mix and match your SWOT data to discover the most potent intersections in light of what you have versus what you need and what is now possible versus what you have already achieved. Examples are key strengths matched with assets to meet challenges, a lesson learned crossbred with a weakness, a weakness married to an opportunity to generate a skill or nourish a relationship (colleague, new hire, mentor). Hitching a weakness to an advantage, a resource, or an opportunity transforms the problem of your weakness into a strategy worth investigating.

The best way to figure out the strategies to resolve your critical issues is with the exercise below. Prevent headaches and wasted resources (such as time and money) later by generating your best strategies now. Now is *not* the time to aim for a solid B–. Now *is* the time to sharpen your thinking axe and fire up the laser of your mind into a peak state. I find that a good night's sleep, early morning cold shower, contemporary piano playlist, and double-shot cappuccino help. As you lean into your critical issues, tune your presence of mind to notice a flash of insight. Trust the process. Let it evolve the way you think to build dynamic synergies that plow the path forward.

Generating Your Strategies from Critical Issues

The time required for this exercise varies between an hour or two and a full day, or perhaps over the course of a week, depending on your level of commitment to your vision. Return to this exercise annually as part of your planning for yourself, your family, and your work. Also, you can return to it whenever you hit a roadblock later.

1. Review your three-year vision and your SWOT data. Your first aim is to convert the most relevant issues you should be focused on—the big guns you circled in your SWOT data—into questions.

2. Play with the possibilities. Account for the *most* relevant issues and opportunities, which showed up in your SWOT data, with a series of "How might I . . .?" questions. Aim for around four to seven critical questions. What strengths could you pair with a crucial weakness or lack of skill? What resources could you shuttle into an opportunity? What are the biggest threats that need to be matched with assets, relationships, or strengths from your data? That is how you want to play the mix-and-match strategy game. For example, if my goal were to write my first book, a critical question might be: How might I leverage my twenty years' experience in my field (strength) with my five years

of blogging experience (strength) and my friend's expertise as a book editor (relationship) with my lack of experience in writing a book (weakness)?

3. Refine your four to seven critical questions down to three clear, concise, and specific questions. If you are having trouble narrowing down to three, see if you can mix and match strengths and opportunities a bit more. Chisel your most pressing issues and opportunities into something useful to bring your strategies into plain view.

4. Now comes the fun part of turning your questions into strategies. Rewrite your three critical questions into three statements by dropping the "How might I . . ." and adding an action-provoking verb. Examples of action verbs are *alchemize, amplify, engage, gather, leverage, magnify, maximize, uplevel*. Rewrite your questions into three strategies. For example, if my goal were to write my first book, my strategy becomes: *Leverage my twenty years' experience in my field (strength) with my five years of blogging experience (strength) and talk to my friend about hiring her as a book editor (relationship) to coach me through writing a great book (weakness).*

5. Are your three strategies addressing the most probable issues that could keep you from your three-year vision? Confirm by making sure your strategies

   • combine your biggest strengths, resources, assets, competencies, opportunities, relationships, threats, and weaknesses.

   • inspire action with a vital verb.

   • directly address your most critical issues.

That's it. Your strategies are the north star for your three-year vision. Your strategies emerged from tapas, the friction of evolution, and resonate with tejas, inspired illumination. You will be so glad you invested your mental fire up front to light a smart path forward. To follow through with the book example above, I can now investigate what I want to pull from my twenty years' experience in a niche, researching which blog posts have been the most popular, and hiring a book writing coach. Later, when unforeseen challenges arise or doubt creeps in, I'll be better prepared to stay the course knowing I formulated strategies based on my real issues. ■

One-Year Milestones

In a short story by Haruki Murakami, the protagonist, a young man, reflects on what an older gentleman taught him: "Your brain is made to think about difficult things. To help you get to a point where you understand something that you didn't at first. And that becomes the cream of your life. The rest is boring and worthless."[13] Mental focus is rare in the short attention span of modern culture. Fire element engages difficult thinking. If you've been doing the exercises up to this point, and you've processed your vision and your critical issues into the most effective strategies, you can set milestones for a year and perhaps longer.

Rock cairns on ancient paths informed our ancestors when they'd arrived at a destination. These stacked stones—or milestones—still serve as landmarks with which to orient oneself. In this section, we'll create milestones to serve as SMART goals for the journey. SMART stands for specific, measurable, actionable, realistic, and timebound. Following these as if they were a stack of rocks marking miles on the trail, you can reach the point where you want to be at a certain time.

Now comes the straightforward part. For each strategy you've identified, you get to ask yourself: "What could I accomplish this year?" Using the example above, I could gather my most popular blog posts; hire a book coach to help with an outline and a time line and advise me on writing books versus blogs; and aim for a rough manuscript in a year. My strategy is turning into an action plan, and even next season's best route is becoming visible.

What could you feasibly accomplish in one year from today? Work your three strategies into one-year milestones: three big, specific, one-year outcomes that will lead to your three-year vision.

You are outlining your plan for the year—your annual plan—by identifying three one-year milestones. Check that your milestones are SMART; for example, in my case, a 60,000-word, first-draft manuscript based upon my most popular writing completed within one year.

Then, check that your milestones resonate with all five bodies (refer to chapter 5 for the Five-Bodies Check-in). If what you've written seems too big, it probably is. Customize it so it feels right spiritually, intuitively, mentally and emotionally, energetically, and physically.

Seasonal Milestones and Your Action Plan

Imagine it's twelve weeks from now. Ask yourself: "What might I have easily accomplished in the first twelve weeks of working toward my annual milestones?" These are the specific mile markers you want to hit this season, confident and surefooted. You are becoming a master of fire, churning vision into reality. Your next task is to find the essential seasonal milestones you want in the next twelve weeks and the action plan to go along with them.

1. Review your annual milestones to find how best to set up the first leg of the journey. What is the best work to do in the season ahead? Try writing *in the past tense* a quick list of results, as if you already accomplished them (e.g., "I completed the book outline and received feedback from three people").

2. Finalize a short list of SMART milestones due in twelve weeks—at least one for each annual milestone.

3. Track your seasonal milestones on a spreadsheet or a free project-management tool, such as Asana, Trello, or Basecamp (which offer free versions and video training on project planning).

4. Break your seasonal milestones into specific to-dos either month by month or week by week. Write each to-do with an action verb. Be specific so it's clear when you can mark each one as done. This is your seasonal action plan, and your list will be unique to your annual milestones, your seasonal milestones, and what's realistic for you.

5. Each season you'll want to review your annual milestones and repeat this quick process (see Figure 6.1).

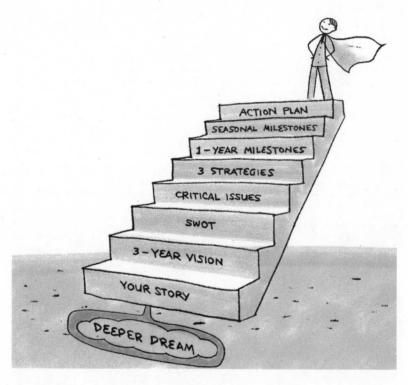

Figure 6.1 Your three-year vision is rooted in your deeper dreams and your story, and the strategies for your milestones rely on your SWOT and critical issues, which will lead you to your action plan.

Use this worksheet to finalize your findings with the fire element exercises. You can print copies of this worksheet from masterofyou.us/workbook.

Three-Year Vision Statement	Strengths	Weaknesses	Opportunities	Threats

Critical Issues	Three Strategies	One-Year Milestones	Seasonal Milestones	Seasonal Action Plan
1	1	1	1	1
				2
2	2	2	2	3
				4
				5
3	3	3	3	6
				7
				8
				9
				10

You're building a trail across uncharted terrain. This process, done iteratively, builds strong neural pathways. But the first pass on the trail is rough. With heavy usage, the trail becomes natural, fluid, and familiar. My first pass through this unfamiliar terrain of vision into action was a mental struggle. Over time, I developed mental capacities with fire, and you will too. As with all the elements, mastering fire will serve you incalculably in coming years. You'll turn vision into reality faster and truer to you than you ever thought possible. This seasonal planning process dovetails with the change of seasons and with regularly updating your home environment (space element) to work for you. As the seasons change, the atmosphere outside stimulates an ancient internal desire to focus on what is coming and to reflect on what you want to do next. Tune in to the change of seasons, and notice your awareness shift out of a ground-level view of life and into an eagle-eye perspective. Ride this momentum to refresh your home and your habits and to set your next season's milestones. The Master of You process gives you a chance to step out of the ordinary, to pull back the arrow, and to point your shakti with greater accuracy toward dharma.

You'll want to revisit your story, three-year vision, SWOT, critical issues, strategies, and annual milestones. Create an annual ritual—a special day or weekend—to set yourself up right for the coming year. For my family's annual planning session, we have casual conversations a few weeks before and schedule a special day to work the exercises and formalize our annual and next season's milestones. I pass on this core life skill to my daughter, as natural as spring cleaning the house, for her to lead her future strategically. I'm proud to report that she hits her seasonal and annual milestones consistently. Because she has done the work to make her milestones clear, it's easy to support her dreams.

Your vision comes to fruition season by season. Every twelve weeks, schedule a few hours to plan your seasonal milestones and outline your next twelve weeks in a spreadsheet or project-management tool. Harness the power of seasonal transitions. Although demanding mental sharpness and periods of concentrated effort, this process becomes natural and fluid. This is the tapas that generates tejas—the illumination of spirit. Now that your vision is embedded in next season's action plan, it's time to master time—air element.

MASTER OF FIRE (AMBITION)

◯ You are a visionary regarding your own life. You invest in yourself by developing a three-year vision that resonates with all parts of yourself.

◯ You approach your critical issues as evolutionary adventures in making your vision happen.

◯ You digest your critical issues into success strategies.

◯ You set specific annual and seasonal milestones rooted in your strategies.

◯ You are able to radically evolve your identity to meet the needs of your three-year vision.

◯ You repeatedly expand beyond who you have already been.

◯ You author your life.

7

AIR: MASTER OF TIME

Now is the time to enter the unconstrained, playful realm of air element. Air element is responsible for all movement and rhythm, including time. In air element, you allow your time to be shaped by your dharma, now embedded in your annual and seasonal milestones.

In mastering air element, you will shape-shift your time, your calendar, to manifest your seasonal milestones. You'll structure the hours of your week to experience flow, focus, and freedom. You'll uncover what you need to stop doing and what could be delegated to free up time. The master of air is full of possibility and thinking outside the box.

Air element, also known as *vayu*, or wind, in Ayurveda, is movement across space. To understand the relationship of air element with time, let's momentarily turn back to air's partner, space element. You'll recall that space's main quality is expansion, or movement without a direction. Space, in its omnipresent quality, expands faster than light moves.[1] Expansion creates space, and then air moves directionally through that space. Conceptually, movement across distance creates the measurement of time, such as the time it takes the wind to cross the valley. Similarly, the distance between heavenly bodies is measured in time—in light years, minutes, and seconds. Light travels the distance from the moon to our eyes in about one second, which means the moon is about one light second away. Sunlight takes about eight minutes to reach our eyes, so the sun is about eight light minutes away.[2] We measure time in cycles:

a day is the time it takes the earth to spin once around; a year is the time the earth takes to loop around the sun. In this chapter, you'll connect the freedom and momentum of air element with the concept of time and the seasons measuring your movement toward your milestones.

Air element is characterized by multidirectional mobility as well as lightness, dryness, subtlety, and spontaneity. The direction of the other elements is predictable: space expands without direction, fire rises, and water and earth descend because of their mass and the gravitational force of the planet. Moving air transfers water from the oceans into clouds, spreads wildfires, and spins tornadoes. Conceptually, the mental-emotional qualities of air element are curiosity, enthusiasm, and abstract or out-of-the-box thinking. Later in this chapter, you'll apply these qualities to innovate your schedule, the way you invest your time.

You can "wind-tunnel" your time. When air moves through a tunnel or spins into a shape like that of a hurricane, the structure or shape builds force. When your time is structured wisely toward your milestones, you gain momentum. How you structure your time precedes your evolution with time management. The better you structure your calendar, the easier it is to manifest your milestones.

The more jurisdiction you have over your time, the less stress you experience and the freer and more empowered you become.[3] Your time is your life. In mastering time, you reshape your habits using your daily and weekly calendar to steer directly toward your milestones, which reflect your vision. When both your direction and your speed are in a natural rhythm, you experience flow. To investigate this, notice how you feel about the week ahead. Are you at ease or overwhelmed? Is your scheduled time aligned to your milestones? You'll feel happiest when you have the right mix of aligned action and free time in your calendar for focus and flexibility to allow for exploration and spontaneity.

According to Ayurveda, air element in the body is disturbed by hurrying and scurrying and being overscheduled. This turns into stressed-out emotional overwhelm and eventual breakdown of the immune system. From mastering earth, you know the connection between arrhythmic living and compounding stress. The American Psychological Association found in its Stress in America online survey that 75 percent of Americans reported that their stress levels are so high they feel unhealthy, with one-third of parents reporting that their stress levels are extreme.[4] Much stress is caused by people taking work home or always being "on call" via email and phone, which disrupts leisure and family time, wears on the nervous and endocrine systems, and eventually affects the immune system. The Mayo Clinic states, "The long-term activation of the stress-response system—and the subsequent overexposure to cortisol and other stress hormones—can disrupt almost all your body's processes, including anxiety, depression, digestive problems, headaches, heart disease, sleep problems, weight gain, and memory and concentration impairment."[5]

Clearly, you don't want to rush around packing more into your days to make your milestones. Rhythm must synchronize your daily schedule and calendar. Mindfulness practices, which make you more aware of the present moment, including meditation, contemplation, and pranayama, also shift the subjective experience of time.[6] When you bookend your days with a breath-centered practice, you shift your subjective experience to what feels like time slowing down, tapping into the relaxation response and regaining control of your time. You shape-shift your time to evolve who you are.

If you've been reading this book sequentially, you have some mindfulness practices in your toolkit from these exercises: Adopt a Cosmocentric Viewpoint (chapter 3), Expand Your Inner Space (chapter 4), the Five-Bodies Check-in (chapter 5), and the WHO Breath (chapter 5). Now let's take those a step further and practice slowing the breath to slow down time.

MEASURE TIME IN BREATH CYCLES

The yogis of yore measured their lifetime on earth in breaths, not in years.[7] Yogis still practice *pranayama*, or slow deep-breathing practices, to lengthen their breath cycles. The ancient yogis observed that this slowed the process of aging. Today, studies on morning breathing practices show the same results: prolonged life span in a range of people, from the general population to those with cancer.[8] In addition to extending longevity, slow diaphragmatic breathing awakens mindfulness and converts the stress response into the relaxation response. The yogis use breathing practices to access higher states of consciousness beyond the ordinary mind—kosha, or the spiritual body. From this relaxed and expansive vantage point, subjective time slows down.

The experience of breathing slowly and deeply is like seeing the whirlwind from a still point or being in the calm eye of the hurricane. This perspective opens the door to aligned action. You can witness your thoughts and gain control over your racing mind—or becoming mindful. When you're consciously relaxed, you are recharging. Your immune system is recovering and growing resilient. Your body also relaxes, slowing biological aging; your mind can focus, your endocrine system (hormones) rebalances, and your cells get more oxygen to decrease inflammation.[9] With more space between thoughts and with a slower respiratory rate, which leads to a slower heart rate, you access ease and focus.

The opposite—shallow, rapid, unconscious breathing—makes for lousy concentration and compromised decision making. You not only speed up your perception of time but also you generate more busyness. Like increases like: being overscheduled and overwhelmed reinforces the pattern, increasing the risk of immune and endocrine problems. Shallow breathing accelerates other aging markers, reflected in increased blood pressure, a faster heart rate, a higher respiratory rate, and stress hormone production.[10] Chronic stress leads to poor decisions, including how to manage your time.

Start your morning with a deep-breathing practice to expand your perspective of time and open up the potential of the day ahead. Try the exercise below.

Slow Your Breath to Slow Down Time

(You can also listen to an audio recording of this exercise at masterofyou.us/workbook.)

Set a timer for two minutes. To open possibilities regarding time, turn your attention inward toward your breath. Sit up tall, on the edge of your seat. Exhale slowly, completely, and gently. Pause. Inhale slowly and completely, without expending too much effort.

Notice that as you exhale, the universe of you contracts. As you inhale, the universe of you expands. The contraction-expansion cycle generates rhythm. Drop into the slower rhythm. In your rhythmic breathing, notice the play between consciousness and time. Relax into your rhythm of slower breathing until your timer goes off. Notice if your perspective of time ahead in your day or night has changed. Notice if you have more awareness of your thinking, of your choices, of what to do next. ∎

When you experiment with time and consciousness by slowing your breath, you open your awareness to higher efficiencies. As you develop a deeper level of mindfulness, you witness your thoughts. You might expose outdated thinking and habits that waste your time. Certain ways you spend time will no longer seem appropriate. For example, Master of You course members often prioritize waking up earlier, trading in evening alcohol, overeating, and screen time for setting up the next day for success. Through slowing down with rhythmic living and aligning distraction-free spaces with your deeper dreams, you can trigger the habits you want to make automatic, from flossing to bookending your day with breathing practices. Although this might sound reasonable yet strait-laced, your deeper dreams become so much more exciting than pinot noir and the newest TV series.

With your breath, you practice metaphorically giving air a structure, exhaling more deeply to inhale more expansively. You contract to expand. The same goes for time. Your calendar, or how you invest your time, is the key to structuring your time to your seasonal milestones.

Master Your Constitution: Learn Your Dosha

Each of the three constitutions can have a different approach to the exercises with time. Pittas, because of their mental focus and natural ability with managing time and projects, should follow their desire to quickly apply these exercises. Kaphas, who tend to flow with time, might approach this process with curiosity about optimizing their time

→

to experience more joy in the process of gliding toward their goals. Vatas might find that their love of spontaneity can be disruptive to managing their milestones; however, they might find in future iterations that time and project management themselves are worthy milestones.

OPTIMIZING YOUR CALENDAR AS A SPIRITUAL PRACTICE

Big questions arise as you schedule your milestones into your life and as you attempt to do what you say you'll do. As Jordan B. Peterson advises, "Act on what you say, so you can find out what happens. Then pay attention."[11] Acting on your milestones sets you up for your next evolution by changing your calendar.

Restructuring your calendar to support your milestones bolsters your spiritual growth. Your dharma requires time management to achieve your vision. This is hard to do at first but with practice becomes natural. The practice is making big or small decisions that prioritize the new identity emerging from your past identity. This includes skillfully blocking out time for your evolving needs. Syncing your schedule to support your body rhythms leads to increased states of focus, productivity, and rejuvenation. Seen in this light, prioritizing your milestones in your schedule and having integrity with what you put on your calendar become body, mind, and spiritual practices.

To support your spirit, you also want your time to be productive and playful, structured and unstructured, efficient and spontaneous. For now, call to mind the playful, light, free-moving, curious, and refreshing qualities of air to open your perspective. Scheduling in playful, free time is essential to pulse the spanda in the opposite direction from structured productivity. Air element is paradoxical. This is the black and white of the yin and yang. Freedom and boundaries are the essential pulsation, the dynamic opposites, which generate synergies otherwise not possible. Air changes both direction and speed, vitalizing spirit with spontaneity. To experience the speed of productivity that happens with better structure, as in a wind tunnel, you also want to allow completely unstructured time to explore new territory.

Next, you'll make an innovative calendar—one that steers you directly toward your current desires regarding your milestones and honors your spirit. My first innovative calendar was a pipedream—entirely out of reach. But I recalled Peterson's words: "Note your errors. Articulate them. Strive to correct them. That is how you discover the meaning of your life."[12] By trying to align my calendar to my vision, I opened my mind to new thoughts that served as guideposts for better daily decisions. When I repeated this iterative exercise over the years and learned along the way, my spiritual practice of aligning purposeful milestones became my weekly calendar. Master of You course members have also found that their subconscious minds find opportunities to implement their innovative calendars with small choices or huge overhauls. Depending on where you are now—how far apart your innovative calendar is from your real calendar—it might take many seasons, maybe years, yet you'll find everyday opportunities to make it real.

This next creative exercise can provoke incremental changes or even a great leap forward with your real calendar. Let's get time on your side.

Your Innovative Calendar

Schedule twenty to sixty minutes to do this exercise. It is a liminal thinking exercise—beyond the threshold of the conditioned mind—to discover how you'd like to live your next month or season. You'll see what you *dream* on paper (or in your online calendar) in order to stimulate your ideas and build your skills with creative time management.

To prepare, you'll need a blank calendar and a fresh mind. If you use an online calendar, such as Google Calendar, create a new, blank calendar. If you use a paper calendar, use a blank monthly calendar for the month ahead.

1. Open your blank calendar.

2. Read aloud your three-year vision and your next season's milestones. Attune to your five

bodies. Tune in to the spirit of possibility: you can have jurisdiction over your time.

3. Schedule your body rhythm habits of nourishing yourself, moving, and sleeping. Be realistic and efficient.

4. Next, what needs to happen each week to hit your milestones? How might you schedule blocks of time to act on your milestones?

5. Imagine you can use the remaining time however you would like. What else do you schedule? You are intentionally leaving aside existing commitments and awakening your deeper desires about time.

6. If you made your calendar online, print it out. Look over your new, innovative calendar. Absorb what you would do if you had full jurisdiction over your time. Do a quick Five-Bodies Check-in to confirm that your innovative calendar resonates fully with all of your bodies.

7. Tape your calendar to your bathroom mirror so you can read it daily. Read it with an open mind.

8. Do this exercise seasonally, riding the change in atmosphere, when you set your milestones. With repetition come big results.

That's it. Relax, exhale, and absorb your innovative calendar in your cells. You have steered your attention, like a wind tunnel captures the movement of air, to what you're aiming for—to what your body, mind, and spirit want. You know your ideal. ■

Attune to the Ayurvedic Clock

The doshas, energies derived from the elements, also cycle through the daily circadian rhythm. The time before dawn (vata time) is dominated by space and air, making it a great time of day for clear thinking and bigger visions. This is a good time of day to meditate. After the sun rises (kapha time), earth and water elements dominate, giving strength to the body. This is the best time to work out and to tackle big projects that need deep focus or very physical projects. By midday, when the sun is brightest (pitta time), fire dominates and bile rises—making it the best time for digestion—so eat your biggest meal then. The energy returns in the afternoon to space and air (vata time), making that time great for communication, management, and planning activities. As the day gives way to night (kapha time), earth and water descend to create a cozy, relaxed, social end of the day. This is why Ayurveda recommends winding down well before 10:00 p.m. After 10:00 p.m. through after midnight (pitta time), fire is active again, doing the intense job of cleaning house. If you are asleep, this fire detoxes and refreshes your system like a forest fire making way for new growth. The cycle begins again with space and air before the dawn (vata time).

STRUCTURE TIME FOR PERSONAL EVOLUTION

To reconcile your innovative calendar with what you have going on next week, let's talk about structuring time. Creating your calendar with time blocks gives shape and control to your weekly schedule. Dan Sullivan at Strategic Coach advises structuring time into free days (free of work and obligations), focus days, and buffer days. Free days replenish your body, mind, and spirit for the heavy lifting of focus and buffer days.[13] Buffer days are for completing the activities that interrupt your deep focus. Activities for buffer days include communication, research, project management, and planning. Focus days allow for uninterrupted time to concentrate on the projects required to reach your milestones. Focus days move hard projects forward at light speed.

Having free, buffer, and focus days on your calendar each week might seem like a pipedream. When I first heard of this, I couldn't imagine making it happen. After years of engaging time as a spiritual practice, I live by it. The way I transitioned was through thinking big and testing small. Often you can't restructure an entire day, but you can structure part of a day—a time block. I started with the advice of Brian Moran, author of *The 12 Week Year*, by structuring strategic blocks, buffer blocks, and breakout blocks into one day.[14] Strategic blocks are like Sullivan's focus days. Buffer blocks are like Sullivan's buffer days, and breakout blocks are equivalent to free time, or a period when you get out of the "office."

Where to begin? Start by restructuring your current calendar. If you have a job or are self-employed, find focus blocks and buffer blocks in your work schedule. The goal is to stop bouncing between activities, a proven stress builder. See where you can restructure your time at work to be more productive and less interrupted. Consider where and when you best focus and where and when you best buffer. Talk with your supervisor, or if you are self-employed, talk with a colleague or a coach about how you'd like to structure your time for greater productivity without stress. If you are paid based on hours and not performance, consider restructuring your contract based on goals your supervisor sets for you or that you set together. To access time freedom and creative freedom, you want to be motivated based on your goals and accomplishments, not just based on showing up. If your work is inflexible with no way to leverage your time, you might consider creating a personal milestone to seek contract work or projects that help you contribute your best work and experience more time freedom.

A new Master of You online course member began the program very overwhelmed. She had three school-aged children, a professional managerial job, and a lifelong struggle with obesity. As she grasped the importance of body rhythms, she wanted to radically restructure her schedule at home and at work. Her supervisor valued her contributions and wanted her to be healthier and happier so she could be a better leader while still putting in the same number of hours at the office. They agreed she could arrive earlier and clock out earlier, allowing her to pick up her kids from school and eat an earlier dinner. She began losing weight and getting more sleep. Gaining momentum with her milestones, she chose to wake up even earlier to exercise before work. Her supervisor noticed she was healthier, happier, and more productive. This motivated her to continue to tweak how she structured her time to meet her personal milestones, her family's needs, and her professional goals.

After five years of seasonal shifts in my calendar, it looks like this: Monday and half of Tuesday are buffer days: meetings, interviews, networking, delegating projects, readying projects for focus days. Tuesday's other half, Wednesday, and Thursday are focus days to hit milestones (including writing, coaching, and running the company). If I finish everything by Thursday, I take Friday off. Otherwise Friday is a focus day. My global online team is on a similar schedule because our priority is to focus to make our milestones. Some of our focus time involves collaborative working sessions. As a team, on buffer days, we get what we need from each other for focus days.

Notice where in your life you have the freedom to innovate with your time. Point your awareness toward what is malleable within your current structured and unstructured time. As needed, review the ethos in chapter 3 to align your mindset to one of experimentation. Work with this structure, and like your breath, you'll be able to slow down time to meet your milestones. As the cliché goes, with iteration and failing fast, the "impossible" becomes *I'm possible*.

Whatever upholds the essence of your milestones is crucial. Just as space freedom requires removing the unessential objects, time freedom requires continually removing the unessential activities. This constant attention to pruning done right generates new growth. To prune a tree, you cut certain limbs and random baby shoots sucking energy from the trunk. Pruning is streamlining resources for growth. Step back seasonally to see your calendar objectively in light of the next season's milestones. Then, update your innovative calendar to align with who you are now and what you want next. Riding the change of weather with the seasonal shifts is a powerful practice that invites you to change and grow. With each iteration, you'll spot what must go for these milestones to be possible. If how you spend your time hasn't been evolving, you have to do a lot of pruning. Do the exercise below to find out what is no longer essential.

What I No Longer Want to Do

First, reread your milestones, and open your innovative and current calendars. Then, ask yourself the questions below. List each time-consuming activity on a line. (You can download and print this worksheet from masterofyou.us/workbook.)

1. What can I delete? What could I just stop doing that is not the best use of my time?

2. What do I no longer want to do that someone else could do?

3. What skills are required?

4. What is the hourly rate for these skills?

5. Who do I know that is qualified? Who could I pay or barter with for that skill?

What I No Longer Want to Do	Skills Required	Hourly Rate for These Skills	Who Do I Know That Is Qualified?

Every time you do this, you will realize more ways to grow your time.

Over the years, I've delegated housekeeping, home projects, yardwork, bookkeeping, errands, dropping off the recycling, grocery shopping, technical computer work, copyediting, and other people's laundry to family and people online or living locally whom I contract for help. The youngest contractor I've hired is my neighbor, who is great at helping me spring clean, put together swag kits for Yogahealer.com events, and reorganize my workspace. Each of our lists will be unique and will change over time. You might love grocery shopping but not carpooling. As you fill in the worksheet, notice which conversations you need to have next. Are you cooking all the meals and doing all the shopping? Do other family members need to pick up slack? Do you need to find a neighbor kid or a skilled contractor?

Bartering is another great option for handing off what you no longer want to do and investing your energy in your milestones without spending money. I've grown my time on the yogic tradition of barter. For example, a local yoga or Ayurveda student might help me with household and career tasks, from cleaning and cooking to preparing herbal formulas, in exchange for courses and teaching. I did the same when I was a yoga student. In my online courses, advanced members trade mentoring new members in exchange for ongoing community access. Do you have a skill that leverages your time that you could use for barter? Pooling resources is another way that people open up time. Joining a neighborhood soup club, trading day care, and carpooling are common examples. Clear contracts stating what will be exchanged by when and what is expected are essential for bartering. Be sure to revisit and renew the agreement if expectations change. When you put your mind to it, you can free up vast blocks of time to focus on your seasonal milestones. ▪

MASTER OF CALENDAR INTEGRITY

As Jocko Willink, commander of the most decorated special ops unit of the Iraq War and a US Navy Seal for twenty years, emphatically points out, *discipline equals freedom*. Willink states, "If you want more free time, you have to follow a more disciplined time management system."[15] Each day you can run experiments with your time: What will you do when? What will you delete, delegate, or do yourself? What do you want to do in your unstructured time? "Time magnifies the margin between success and failure. It will multiply whatever you feed it. Good habits make time your ally. Bad habits make time your enemy," writes habit master James Clear.[16]

Say your milestone is to write the first draft of a book outline. You schedule time in your calendar for writing between 6:00 and 7:00 a.m. five days a week. If you have integrity with yourself and your calendar, you no longer decide if you're going to write that day. You built your decision into your structure. Calendar integrity becomes a goal in itself to unleash your power over time. You reduce the likelihood of staying up too late, checking your phone when you wake up, or whatever normally keeps you from writing between 6:00 and 7:00 a.m. Additionally, you might stop watching Netflix at night as you build momentum with your milestone and find yourself going to bed earlier and waking earlier, proven habits for peak performance.

Time measures progress objectively. Either you get closer to your milestones or you don't. Just as accountants regularly reconcile accounts, masters of time reconcile their milestones with their calendar and to-do list or with a project-management tool.

Alignment Meetings

(To print copies of the worksheet for your meetings, go to masterofyou.us/workbook.)

Schedule a twenty-minute weekly meeting with yourself during a buffer block to reconcile your next week with your milestones. You've laid some great groundwork to better structure your time. To keep yourself on track with your innovative calendar and your seasonal milestones week after week, use the four Rs: Ready, Review, Reorganize, Reaffirm.

Ready: Set a timer for twenty minutes. Open your calendar, your seasonal milestones, your innovative calendar, and your What I No Longer Want to Do worksheet.

Review: Review your seasonal milestones and next week's calendar. Review your ideal, or innovative, calendar. You might have made some progress. Review what you've accomplished on your milestones or ideal calendar and what you can accomplish this week. Use the four questions of problem-solving from a school of thought called design thinking: What is working? What isn't working? Why is it not working? What is the biggest challenge? The purpose is to get an honest snapshot of your evolution with time.

Reorganize: Based on your current biggest challenge with your milestones and your calendar, take a moment to pause. What do you need to say no to next week to say yes to your milestones? For example, for me to write this book, I have to say no to reading fiction. Fiction to me is like Netflix series are to others. I'm also saying no to any alcohol for clearer thinking. I'm saying yes to going to bed by 9:30 p.m. every night and writing before dawn most days. Each week, think big in terms of your seasonal milestones and test small by upgrading what you say no and yes to.

Reaffirm: When your timer goes off, take a moment to reflect, recognize, and reaffirm your identity evolution over time. Absorb your progress. Affirm what is working in your evolving calendar. ■

ALIGNMENT MEETINGS AS A GROUP

When your milestones involve other people, try a weekly or bimonthly meeting with the above process. Most of my milestones are entwined with those of family and Yogahealer.com team members. As you grow your ambitions, you'll notice more people are involved. Alignment meetings build a clarified momentum for our week ahead. By carving out a brief time weekly to plan the week ahead and resolve any conflicts that arose over the previous week, you can prevent small problems from developing into big ones. For instance, in a family alignment meeting, if one person needs extra support in food preparation or parenting that week for the family to run smoothly, this is the right time to ask for that support and rearrange the schedule. If a family or team member seems out of alignment with the group's ethos, this is the best time to discuss it and get realigned.

For example, you don't want to throw a jab at someone while preparing dinner for not pulling their weight. Set a time and place weekly to discuss these values and realign. Asking for specific support ahead of time is easier than asking on the fly. With my husband, when one of us has a big week ahead, the other is able to realign ahead of time, which prevents stress and crises. Rather than getting sucked backward by a daily rhythm that is no longer highly functional, you want to leverage your newly developing strengths together.

Use alignment meetings for any group of people (a family, project team, mastermind group, partnership) that shares milestones and calendars. Alignment meetings reinforce what is working and what must shift. At work and at home, alignment meetings bring to the surface and resolve scheduling issues, communication issues, behavioral issues, and discrepancies between ethos and habits—between reality and the dream.

In an alignment meeting, members know why they are needed there, their desired outcomes, the agenda, and the time frame. The agenda should reflect the group's ethos. The time frame for families is shorter: fifteen to thirty-five minutes is usually sufficient. With teams, thirty to sixty minutes might be appropriate. Emphasize goals, learning, habits, schedules, and support. Choose some of the questions below to generate an agenda together or create your own.

1. What is the progress on our milestones?

2. What outcomes do we want for today's meeting?

3. What are you looking to accomplish this week?

4. What did you learn last week?

5. What issues do you want to discuss?

6. What habits will help you reach your goal this week?

7. How can we support you this week?

Often families use a talking stick and work teams use a timer to practice speaking in concise time frames. Equal airtime is important in alignment meetings—where authority does not reign. When we first started having alignment meetings as a family, it was a little too formal and awkward. Now we have our rhythm down, just like you will find yours. Our meetings now spontaneously arise on Sundays at the kitchen table, in the truck, on the chairlift, or in the boat. At our family meetings, we align our priorities, schedules, and even meal plan based on the seasonal changes and our body goals. Yogahealer.com team alignment meetings are more formal, with an updated agenda on a shared document that members have added to during the previous week. We alternate who leads the meetings—at home and work—to build leadership skills.

Side benefits from alignment meetings include giving all members a voice, a supportive audience to speak to, and equal floor time; helping people self-manage their time; and building teamwork skills, meeting skills, and leadership skills. You stop interrupting other people or stop being interrupted by having the wrong conversation at the wrong time (or, in some cases, both). Schedule conflicts, unvoiced expectations, unaddressed behavioral issues, and last-minute discussions about what's for dinner tonight become distant memories. When a new habit, such as a weekly meeting, has side benefits, you know you're on the right track. As a parent or leader, you are underscoring the importance of vision-planning, setting goals, developing good habits, and participating in teamwork in your group.

BEFRIENDING TIME

As you harness the winds of time, you'll notice more acutely when you're out of sync, overwhelmed, breathless, or scurrying about and generating more work, more drama, and maybe even more chaos. You might even feel like you're aging or wearing yourself out faster than you'd like. Feeling out of sync is your cue, your trigger to exhale and have an alignment meeting with yourself to review your annual and seasonal milestones and your calendar and to schedule your rest, habits, and activities for the week ahead. Remember James Clear's words: "Good habits make time your ally."[17]

Befriending air element and time, you gain the power to accelerate or decelerate your pace. You might get the perspective that your identity is evolving at what feels like the speed of light. By taking charge of time, you open to continually improving the experience you want and extending your longevity. You'll also access a timeless, inner quiet that arises when you are calm, centered, and at peace, which we touched on in the previous chapter, on earth element, with sthira (stillness). By experimenting with how you structure time based on your body rhythms, you'll continually gain access to the rhythms of your nature, the spanda—your in-out breath cycles, your focus-free cycles, your rest-digest cycles. As you heed the cycles from a cosmocentric perspective, you might experience your part in a greater rhythm and bigger cycles of evolution. You imprint your three-year vision into the air, the field of time, as it's arising from the blank canvas in front of you.

As you work through this process with your milestones, you improve your ability to track and predict what you can do in a season. Implementing even bits and pieces of these air element exercises can lead to big change over time. You'll become an expert on accurately scoping, planning, and aligning your calendar with your milestones, season by season, which has a compounding positive effect on your potential. This is why some people's lives seem truly ideal, innovative, dreamy, magical, easefully fluid, and yet highly generative. You are actively testing your beliefs about time and how you give direction to air element. The more you tap into the qualities of air—open-minded, light, curious, exploratory—the faster you align to the calendar you want. As you improve, you experience flow—the power of water element—the last but not least element in the Master of You program.

MASTER OF AIR (TIME)

○ You align your body rhythms and your annual and seasonal milestones with your weekly, seasonal, and annual calendar.

○ You schedule blocks of time into free time, focus time, and buffer time for peak performance and deep rejuvenation.

○ You have integrity with your calendar, doing what you say you'll do.

○ You schedule your action steps each week to hit your seasonal milestones.

○ You delete and delegate as a time practice.

○ You have alignment meetings with yourself, your family, and your coworkers to structure the week ahead.

○ You schedule time for planning your seasonal and annual milestones to achieve your three-year vision.

8

WATER: MASTER OF INTEGRITY AND FLOW

At long last, we arrive at water element. With the Master of You program, you become master of your dharma and your possibilities for a more capable you. Reflect on how you have evolved your space, your body rhythms, your ambitions, and your time. Are you collaborating with the elements to enhance your days? Perhaps you are improving both your resilience and your adaptability: you are supported by your rejuvenating spaces; rooted in your body rhythms; flexible with shaping your calendar according to the skills, competencies, and actions you need to take next to achieve your deeper dreams; and adaptable in becoming who your identity evolution is leading you to become.

You might have found, arriving here in water element, that at many points in this journey tough challenges, frustration, and discouragement have surfaced. Perhaps unanticipated setbacks arose. In acting on purposeful ambitions, you provoked purposeful challenges. Such challenges might have edged your seasonal or annual milestones out of reach and might be testing you at your core. Fascinatingly, this is how the game of mastery works. Adaptability will be essential, and its lesson is best taught by water. This lesson is almost as old as time; it is described in the classic sixth-century *Tao Te Ching*: "Water is fluid, soft, and yielding. But water will wear away rock, which is rigid and cannot yield. As a rule, whatever is fluid, soft, and yielding will overcome whatever is rigid and hard. This is another paradox: what is soft is strong."[1]

To rise to greater heights, you will first be escorted to your depths—or what depth psychologists describe as the unconscious or semiconscious mental processes, or the shadows, and their motives, often related to what you might have repressed, rejected, denied, or ignored.[2] The original depth psychologists, including Carl Jung, Sigmund Freud, William James, and Pierre Janet, discovered how exploring and processing these underlying motives or patterns is intrinsically healing. Their theories align with ancient myths that reveal how befriending and integrating ineffective or unhealthy patterns create resolution. Obstacles arise when we take action toward our vision. Less evolved patterns, even dysfunctional patterns, will be exposed. This is the feedback we receive and the demand for transformation that must occur if we are to evolve. If we take the feedback and dissolve the outdated pattern, we break through. Such breakthroughs unlock the passage to actualizing your three-year vision. This is the power of water. In this chapter, you will explore the issues that arise in acting on your vision—to heal what needs to be healed and to integrate the next pieces of your personality required to evolve. Stepping into deeper integrity and emotional evolution leads to fluidity in pursuing your dreams.

In water element, you'll turn inward to your challenges rather than away from them, investing your attention in what blocks your way forward, making outdated patterns conscious. Although water element escorts us to our depth, it is also softening, soothing, persistent, and adaptable to the path of least resistance. In Ayurveda, *apas*, or water, is the concept of fluidity, cohesion, protection, and nourishment. Water element softens old patterns within you that must be integrated for you to move forward. Water brings up the hard truth that what got you to this point isn't enough to get you all the way to your three-year vision. In mastering water, you'll explore how what goes wrong (what isn't enough) is actually right. What seemingly goes awry on the journey to your deeper dreams is *necessary* to move forward. This is how water nurtures a more integrated and authentic you.

Undoubtedly, at some point in your heroine's journey, you will encounter the underworld of your dharma—the underbelly of your next purpose—the challenges you need to overcome with your eyes wide open and the essential skills you don't yet have to achieve your vision. When you feel disempowered, caught off guard, or in a territory you didn't enter by choice—when you feel like you were swallowed by a mythological whale—you are in water. Michelle Obama, in her memoir, *Becoming*, describes what yogis could call a "water" moment—the horrible barrage of negative national press in response to speeches she gave in support of her husband's campaign. As campaign advisors intervened, she realized that her skills in speaking to smaller crowds actually worked *against* her with crowds of thousands. Although emotionally the experience was humiliating and demoralizing, she adjusted to her circumstances by advocating for her needs for training, resources, and event management on the campaign trail, stepping up her game in a bigger arena of the public eye.

Why do humans get pulled into their underworld, into the shadows of their subconscious, when seeking a worthwhile goal? When water element swallows you whole, you have a lesson to learn or competency to gain before you can flow forward. Usually the timing is quite inconvenient, halting progress. Most likely, you won't want to engage the lesson at the time and put your plans on hold. Often, there is something you can no longer avoid if you want to move forward. Water element shows up when your next big lesson in life is ripening. If you turn inward, into the now-critical issue, and humbly soften, you open yourself to becoming even more whole and powerful. To circle back to Michelle Obama, months later when her identity shifted to First Lady, she had a new set of skills and was wizened from the campaign trail, ready to devote herself in her new role.

Particularly sticky patterns, or "shadow issues," are deeply repressed, rejected, denied, or hard-to-unpack parts of the self. These patterns make the underworld journey longer and require an attitude of curiosity and receptivity. Yet, after they are transformed, the most growth is possible. As with mastering any element, the obstacles you encounter become easier to face through the iterative exercises, such as the ones included in this chapter. In mastering water, understanding that the underworld is part of navigating the deeper dreams for everyone, including you, will help you generate self-awareness throughout the process. In this chapter, I will help you navigate through tough circumstances with eyes wide open so you can avail yourself of the breakdown that leads to the breakthrough—your next level of integrity, which leads to greater ease, connectedness, and even delight. You will also develop water element traits of self-compassion, healing, replenishment, and adaptability.

In this chapter, you will map your own underworld, releasing yourself from eddies that hold you back from flow. We'll look to mythology for inspiration in orienting ourselves in the underworld of tough times. I'll also share some self-compassion and healing exercises and a quick way to assess the most easeful way forward. As you befriend water, you open the gates to a state of flow in which you access full focus and a sense of capability as you dissolve obstacles and realize your milestones.

Your deeper dreams will churn and bring to the surface what can no longer be out of integrity in you. For the ego, this is often quite uncomfortable at first but is a required piece of the process. As Roman emperor Marcus Aurelius said in *Meditations* in the second century: "The impediment to action advances action. What stands in the way becomes the way."[3]

Explore water element with the following exercise, designed to stir the nourishing powers of water for the journey into your depths and clear the way for flow. Processing the challenges and discouraging situations that arise is the first step in transforming them from negative experiences to lessons learned. By doing so, you gain necessary capacities required for your three-year vision. Use the following exercise to get your cards on the table.

Map Your Underworld and Reckoning Day

Write or sketch your answers to the following questions to get a sense of the stages of your evolutionary underworld journey. (Download the worksheet at masterofyou.us/workbook.)

How is your growth path drawing you into your depth?

What obstacles or challenges are surfacing?

What is out of integrity in your life right now?

What are the integrity gaps, obstacles, or challenges revealing?

What are the emotions that come with these obstacles?

What are you resisting?

In what way are you resisting?

What must be released for the next dimension of you to be born?

How will you surrender your ego for your growth? What patterns, behaviors, and attitudes do you need to surrender? What does surrender look like? What does it feel like?

What actions do you need to take now?

What do you need to learn, and who do you need to become next?

Has your three-year vision changed? If so, how?

Have your one-year milestones changed? If so, how?

Have this season's milestones changed? If so, how?

Do you need to adjust your weekly calendar? If so, how?

Do you need to prioritize one of the body rhythms? If so, how?

How will you know when you've integrated what you need to learn next?

What are the potential outcomes of engaging in this depth work?

In the pit of despair, the darkness obscures the light of your progress. Yet, the pit is a sign you've taken action. You've tried hard enough to fail. After answering these questions, do you know your underworld intimately? Are you more in touch with your critical issues? Do you need to revise your three-year vision, your one-year milestones, your seasonal milestones, or your calendar? If so, know this is normal; you haven't failed, you have learned. You have more information, and being adaptable and resilient, you are navigating a better path forward. ■

THE WEIGHTY, WILY WISDOM OF WATER

As soon as you pursue deeper dreams, outdated patterns surface. As personal as a pattern seems, it's helpful to know that everyone has patterns that surface when they are living a bigger dharma. A pattern will appear as a challenge or a dramatic situation with difficult emotions. Yet the pattern isn't new; it's been there swirling under the surface of your consciousness. The pattern might be generations old, inherited from your ancestors. The situation arising is the gift of water to break down and dissolve the old pattern. Breakdown happens before breakthrough—it's a necessary stage in the identity evolution cycle (see Figure 8.1).

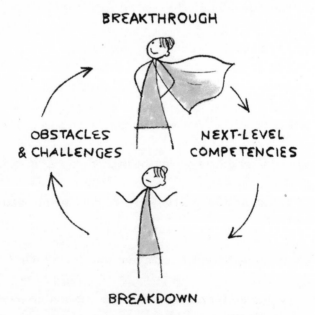

Figure 8.1 Breakdown naturally precedes the breakthrough in the process of identity evolution.

For example, in the Sumerian myth, Inanna willingly goes to the pit of hell in the underworld to gain power from her sister—also queen of the underworld. Inanna dies to her old self in the excruciating process of encountering her own shallow, uncompassionate, power-hungry tendencies. Through layers of humiliations and deaths, she meets her shadow. She can't escape her own outdated identities, which now show up as her inadequacies. She must digest them, layer by layer. When she does, the emotional pain of her incongruencies breaks way to a new level of leadership as queen of the earth and the heavens.

The underworld myths cross cultures and times. Another example is the Greek story of Demeter—known as Mother Nature and the goddess of the harvest and fertility—and her daughter Persephone. The king of the dead abducts the innocent Persephone into the underworld to be his wife. Demeter's sadness over losing her daughter to the underworld sends the earth into winter, halting growth and harvesting. Yet, in the underworld, innocence evolves into awakened power, and Persephone emerges back to the land as queen of the underworld and goddess of spring, of rebirth after death. Persephone, like Inanna, is required to be in the underworld half the year, to return to the darkness, to die to the outside world. The underworld represents the aqueous unknown, the mysterious power that activates the next seasonal cycle of fertility.

From these myths, we learn that the murkiness, the death of the out-dated self, and the grief for that loss are essential for the cycle of growth. Persephone and Inanna represent the root-to-rise concept of spanda (which we explored in chapter 5, on earth element)—both develop hidden powers from their descent, choosing to be queens of darkness in order to be queens of light and life, cycle after cycle. The same spanda—the pulsation—that brings you up also escorts you down. If you go into your own unknown, interested in evolution, your spanda later rebounds with integrated power. The momentum of the descent generates the later ascent, as when you bounce a ball off the floor. The more downward energy, the more upward energy.

You know you are being pulled into water element when your emotions are heavy and overpowering. Fear, frustration, hopelessness, stress, and grief are the gateways to their gravitational opposites of innovation, ease, achievement, optimism, and the delight of integration. By acknowledging your negative emotions and circling through the lessons they hold, you move through the cycle from breakdown to breakthrough, which comes with refined integration of the parts of your self. As Jung pointed out, "No tree, it is said, can grow to heaven unless it's roots reach down to hell."[4]

During a healing or growth journey, we can be pulled under into a disorienting inward abyss of heavy emotions. Time in the abyss itself is disorienting. Often a part of the self feels like it's dissolving or dying, and the sadness can be overwhelming, like Demeter's grief, which stopped growth and harvesting. Yet, remember that the elements, including water, are impersonal—it happens to *everyone* becoming a better version of themselves (see Figure 8.2). The abyss itself is as deep as your ambition is great. Expansion and growth happen through pulsating opposites. What goes up must come down. Root to rise. To jump to great heights, you must bend your knees. As mid-twentieth-century entrepreneur and motivational speaker Earl Shoaff, Jim Rohn's mentor, taught, "Don't wish it were easier; wish you were better."[5]

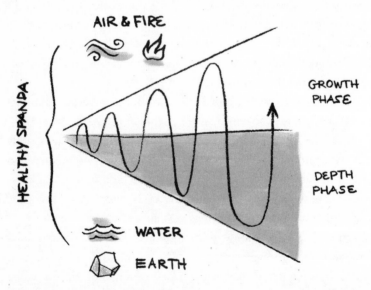

Figure 8.2 Healthy spanda involves cycles of going into an inward and downward depth phase (water) to ascend into a growth phase (air and fire). Any of the breathing practices in this book can help transform the emotional energy from negative to positive: see the Five-Bodies Check-in (chapter 5), the WHO Breath (chapter 5), and the Current in the Box, in this chapter.

I'll share a personal example of my recent integrity gaps. For years I told my mother, who lives a mile away, and my daughter, "I'll play with you more this summer." Yet, for years, I worked as hard during the summer as I did every other time of the year, despite being my own boss. The gap between speech and action was in my integrity. In reflection, I see a past identity tied to not hiring the level of professional help I needed. When I mine my regret, I realize I was holding on too tightly to money, which stressed my mind, body, and core relationships. Integrity gaps bring regret. When mined, regret brings forth gems in the form of lessons learned, or skills or relationships needed, which unfold into an identity evolution. In my case, now that I have professionals working with me, my stress is gone, and I have the quantity and quality of time I want with my child and mother.

Water also swirls in circles. Like an eddy or a whirlpool, this circular motion churns the parts of you that need to evolve next from your subconscious, below the surface of your awareness, into the light of day. My tightfisted, low-overhead business model was depleting all I truly value, but I couldn't see it until the final breakdown before the breakthrough. Although we are all embarrassed by our vulnerabilities and inadequacies, water can help us see and then heal these shadows within ourselves . . . if we can surrender to its wisdom.

The next section and exercise will help you navigate through the murk.

EXCAVATING EASE WITH THE IMPACT-EFFORT GRID

Through every navigable river rapid is a desired route for the whitewater kayaker. The route can be seen as the green water, shaped like a green arrow or tongue, surrounded by the white, troublesome water. The green tongue points the way to the strongest, smoothest, most energetically efficient way forward. As a whitewater paddle boarder, I'm a big fan of finding the green tongue. As with carrying out your ambition, the stakes are high, and opportunities are easily missed because of distraction.

When heading into whitewater, a boater looks for the green water, not the whitewater. If you know the signs of water on a river, it becomes navigable. Whitewater is white because it's mixed with air, showing turbulence, which means trouble.

Where you put your attention, you go—even if that is not where you want to be. Train your eye downstream to spot the green tongue—the desired, efficient path to your seasonal or annual milestones. This unlocks ease, one of the superpowers of mastering water.

The Impact-Effort Grid, from the design-thinking methodology, is a tool to spot the green tongue in whatever rapids arise between you and the milestones of your three-year vision. Use this grid any time, particularly during or after a murky breakdown, when you are questioning what next actions align to the efficient and easeful way through.

Impact-Effort Grid

1. Draw a grid similar to Figure 8.3 (or download the printable version, full instructions, and examples at masterofyou.us/workbook).

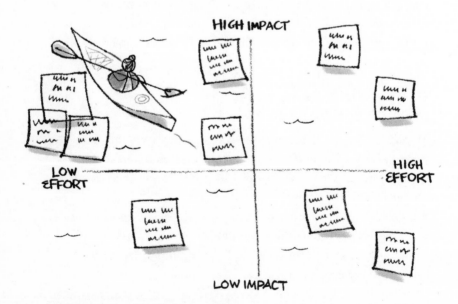

Figure 8.3 Impact-effort grid

2. Choose a challenge you are facing in reaching your milestones, either this season's or this year's. Investigate this challenge by asking: "What is working? What isn't working? What are my biggest challenges? Why isn't it working?"

3. As you digest the challenge with these four questions, ideas for solutions, improvements, and next steps will pop up, like bubbles in water. All ideas are fair game. Write each idea on a sticky note, and then place your sticky notes on the Impact-Effort Grid, determining their placement based on the impact and effort of each. What are the smallest efforts you can make to yield the highest return? For example, say my seasonal milestone is to have a legal living will completed, and the biggest challenge is that I haven't made the time to act. Ideas for solutions might include hiring a lawyer who specializes in wills to manage the project, to set aside time to research and write it myself, to talk to a lawyer friend about which way to go, and to purchase an online living will template. Each of these options goes on a sticky note. How much your time is worth to you influences where you'll put your sticky notes on the Impact-Effort Grid. If you earn $25 an hour, hiring a lawyer is high impact, high effort. If you earn $100 an hour, hiring a lawyer is high impact, low effort. Generating lots of small actions, putting each on its own sticky note, and placing it on the grid will give you a quick cost-benefit analysis of the time and energy you might spend on those actions. You will see which actions have the best return on your effort, and this will affect your investment. That is the green tongue.

4. Choose small actions to test your idea.
    Schedule them for this coming week. Act
    immediately, and notice the green tongue
    revealing the way through the rough water.

This thinking process helps you listen and be in right relationship with your challenge. You refine your route based on reflecting, processing, and transforming your most critical issues into a better plan of immediate action. Make sure to capture not only low-effort, high-impact solutions but also high-effort and much higher-impact solutions by updating your next season's milestones. With practice, you'll become fluid in solving the hardest critical issues. ■

Next, we'll explore self-compassion practices to sustain and invigorate you through mastering water.

SELF-COMPASSION SUPPORTS THE WAY THROUGH WATER

Illogically, we humans fall into a vortex by taking our setbacks personally. Self-blame or self-sabotage for undesired results delay the outcomes you want; the watery emotion of self-compassion is a better way to heal the gap between who you are and who you want to become. Studies in self-compassion, growth mindset, and the benefits of failure clearly point to a better way to approach pressing and chronic issues.

A study on self-compassion focused on first-year students navigating the college transition. Students who reported higher levels of self-compassion felt more optimistic, energetic, and alive during their first semester of college, increasing in tandem their levels of motivation and engagement.[6] Self-compassion enhances the psychological traits of autonomy, competence, and relatedness, which in turn enrich well-being. This self-sufficiency mirrors the yogis' emphasis on shifting your awareness from limitation into potentiality. Engaging issues head-on with self-compassion, honesty, and optimism is the name of the game for lifelong learners on the path to their next breakthrough. Releasing fear or frustration into the healing power of water is self-compassion in action.

Hot Baths

Choose a hot Epsom salt bath to absorb your trauma, your tiredness, your irritation. Add four handfuls of Epsom salts to a hot tub of water. Sprinkle in an essential oil: rose to relax irritation, eucalyptus to deepen your breath, or jasmine to soothe anxiety. Soak. Then wrap yourself in a towel and climb into bed and rest. Investing in relaxation is a potent form of self-compassion.

Cold Showers or Cold Plunges

Doing what helps your body process emotions is self-compassionate, and cold water works wonders to improve circulation and process stuck emotion. According to Ayurveda, many of our unprocessed emotions, including unprocessed ancestral patterns, are stored in *medas dhatu*, or fat tissue, which is dominated by water element.[7] Similar to rhythmic exercise and fasting, showering or bathing in cold water shifts metabolism so that fat (adipose) tissue moves from storage into circulation. This primes the circulation pumps in the interstitial fluid of cells, washing away inflammation and stagnation and improving concentration and optimism.[8]

The result of a few moments a day in cold water? You become more fluid and adaptable, and your immune resilience improves.[9] Modern yogis, notably Wim Hof, along with trending biohackers, reinvigorated this age-old, planetwide custom of cryotherapy (cold therapy). The emerging research from cryotherapy demonstrates success with anti-aging markers and autoimmune healing.

The easiest way to start is with ending your normal shower with cold water. Remember, *think big, test small* with your habit evolution. Build your tolerance and the length of your cold shower or cold plunge slowly, incrementally, and repetitively. Commit and recommit to a daily practice to face the challenges that arise with your dreams. You'll soon enjoy the exhilarating effect, which stimulates relaxation—another example of the pulsation of spanda. Eventually, you might begin each morning with a cold shower. This habit is quite fast to pick up and might quickly become how you start your day to meet the challenges ahead: awake, aware, and resilient.

Below is a practice to wake up your inner energy currents. I use it each morning after my cold shower.

Current in the Box

Like currents flowing downstream, currents of life-force energy run through your body. According to Ayurveda, your body works on a polarity axis from crown to root, which means you have a top and a bottom. As a result of modern culture, most people's energy flows more up than down because our minds are more active and our bodies more stagnant. The breath-body movement described here encourages your body currents to move both up and down as you move your spine like a snake. It awakens your sentient awareness of the wisdom of water within you. Do this exercise to shift your body from stagnant to vibrant, to rebalance your emotions from negative to positive, and to shift your mind from overwhelm into ease. I do this exercise every morning, whether I'm home or on the road. I sometimes will also do it before bed to move any stuck emotions or out-of-alignment vertebrae back into place to rest both energetically clear and physically aligned.

It takes no more than a few minutes. This is a rapid-fire breathing, quick-repetition version of the cat-cow yoga pose—with the exhale on cow (back bend) and the inhale on cat (spine rounded or forward bend). You'll start on all fours, creating a stable position to move energy and invigorate your cells into unified pulsation. Pulse your breath as you move your spine, pumping your cells into a unified pulse, invigorating your body, and clearing your mind. Do it to feel it!

1. Come onto your hands and knees to form a "box" shape. Position your knees under your hips, bottoms of your toes on the floor, spine long, hands under your shoulders, fingers gripping the earth. Push down just enough so they don't move. You have your box; it's time to move your current.

2. Inhale as you reach your nose toward your navel.

3. Exhale as you lift your tailbone and crown of your head toward the sky in opposite directions, as in cow pose.

4. Focus your awareness at the tip of your tailbone and the crown of your head. Inhale, round your back, as in cat pose; exhale and open the front of your body, as in cow pose. Repeat for 20 to 100 breaths to awaken the current and the pulsation of the life force—your shakti. Emphasize exploring the full range of motion in your spine. Find your own pace each day, pumping your body with your breath, slowly at first, and then more quickly as you gain pace. It can be quite fast by the middle or end—unlike in yoga class, which might focus on slower, deeper breathing.

5. Sit back on your heels, with the tops of your feet tucked under you. Absorb the energy you generated through the practice. Feel how energy can move both up and down in your body. Notice the difference so that later in your day, if energy feels stuck or your emotions or thoughts become negative, you can do this again to reregulate yourself.

Now you have another breath-body practice to replenish you through what lies ahead. ■

THE PIT OF DESPAIR, POINT OF NO RETURN, ROCK BOTTOM, AND RECKONING DAY

I'm going to escort you through the territory of what to do when you don't hit your time line, when your critical issues are more critical than expected and seem to breed even more critical issues, and you question your deeper dreams. We often can't accurately judge how long milestones will actually take or what our critical issues actually are. Yet, with iteration of these exercises in vision-planning (fire) coupled with action prioritization (air), we move the needle on creating the reality we want to experience. As serial entrepreneur and author James Altucher advises, "The only truly safe thing you can do is to try over and over again. To go for it, to get rejected, to repeat, to strive, to wish. Without rejection there is no frontier, there is no passion, and there is no magic."[10]

When the going gets tough . . . what happens next? Weaknesses you hadn't identified or realized the scope of during vision-planning (fire) rise to the surface like bubbles out of boiling water when you test your plan. Losing not only energy and momentum but also faith is common in the pit of despair. The circular and at times thickly obscured, cloudy nature of water seems like it isn't evolution at all. But it is. Your evolution took a fast-tracked shortcut through your emotional underworld.

In a few world religions, the day of reckoning refers to the last judgment of God, when after death people have no choice but to account for their actions in life. Reckoning day is the settling of accounts, a no-holds-barred coming to terms with what is, a "come to Jesus" moment in which your cards are on the table, face up. You are facing the truth of who you'll need to become next and what you'll need to transform in yourself to move forward. Or, you can regress into the patterns of your past. This settling of accounts is an honest reassessment of your critical issues. Now is the time to reconsider and adapt, with more intel, who your superheroine is and what she needs to manifest for your three-year vision, your one-year milestones, and your seasonal milestones. This level of depth is the fast path to growth. Ready to face what needs to be faced, you're at the bottom: the shadow is revealed and embraced.

We can learn about water's abyss from childbirth. Birth is an aqueous, messy rite of passage that generally goes better when a woman can surrender to her body leading the way through the process, cooperating with intense expansion of her body as it opens in the largest possible way with the downward current. The true labor of "labor" pulls a woman's consciousness away from the surface. She meets her depth; she unearths the sacred power within her womb. She descends to the netherworld and back to cull forth the heavenly—her child born and herself reborn. So it is with your potential.

In this process of going into and assimilating your depth, water will birth you to a higher, more subtle plane of flow. As you let yourself unravel, you soften deep-seated patterns. Water can then dissolve your patterns, turning you inside out and round and round and escorting you to the surface, back into your growth, as a more integrated, capable, transparent version of yourself. This process removes your obstacles through changing you and your thinking, sometimes as deeply as your beliefs. As I process the old pattern with my promises of time with my mother and my child, I know I can't get that time back. My new identity invests in better help and is careful with time and speech.

You're at the bottom, and you will rebound, which means . . . rebirth, flow, and delight come next!

Master Your Constitution: Learn Your Dosha

Each constitution has different issues with water element. Kaphas might get depressed and lose energy, vatas can get easily overwhelmed, and pittas will get frustrated by the seeming setbacks of water's wily ways. Yet, each dosha type has a special gift in the underworld. If pittas can let go of what they already know and trust water's nonlinear process, their drive and problem-solving abilities will be their asset. Vatas' natural emotional transparency and ability to change quickly will be their asset in water, in that they can build support for themselves in the process. Kaphas' natural ability to go with the flow will be their asset as long as they are very physically active and eat lighter when experiencing the heavier emotions of water.

YOUR BREAKTHROUGH INTO FLOW

The delightful reward of mastering water is the next level of flow, ease, and delight. As a human, you are wired to desire and thrive in a flow state, which maximizes your ability to generate higher levels of self-assessment, skill, challenge, engagement, and connection. As with riding a wave, a master of water learns to move with the pressures of water. This lesson eventually leads to an unwavering state of inner confidence in doing the right thing at the right time, even when the right thing is to pause and reflect for clarification. Mastering your home and office (space), your body rhythms (earth), your vision-planning (fire), your time (air), and integrating your depth (water) will incrementally and at times suddenly deliver you into the relaxed joy of aligned action.

The *flow state*, a term developed and defined by Mihaly Csikszentmihalyi, the psychologist who recognized and named the psychological concept of flow, refers to "being in the zone." He defined flow as "the mental state of operation in which a person performing an activity is fully immersed in a feeling of energized focus, full involvement, and enjoyment in the process of the activity."[11]

Csikszentmihalyi points out that to tap into flow, one needs to strike a balance between the challenge of the task and their own skill. If the task is too difficult or too easy, flow cannot occur. "Too easy" generates boredom, which comes from repetitive tasks in which someone gets stuck in habituated actions, work, or relationships. "Too hard" generates anxiety because the skill level is nowhere near what the challenge demands. For a flow experience, both skill and challenge must be matched at a high level.[12] As you work toward your milestones, your skill level will increase to meet your critical issues. As you encounter the full range of emotions water brings to the surface, you'll reassess your critical issues to meet the challenges, or you'll lessen the challenges as needed. In the iteration of this cycle, you'll become a master of flow—knowing what you can handle. You'll even improve your time-frame estimates for your milestones. With flow, your focus and engagement improve—you begin to trust your desire and your process at unprecedented levels. Flow, like other states, is habit forming. As you build the flow habit, you experience longer states of delight and accomplishment.

FINANCIALLY FLUENT, FLUID, AND ACCUMULATING

As you unleash into flow, better opportunities arise. Opportunities are valuable and tied to an investment of attention, expertise, or money. Some opportunities are directly related to more money—or conducting more currency. Currency represents the flow of value. More currency is in circulation every year. The marketplace is a constantly changing current. Culture and technology continue to spawn new streams with more ways to provide a valuable service or product every moment. Those who collide with currency forget that it's an infinitely expanding value stream, with room for all to play. To become flush with more currency, ask yourself, "What additional value can I add to the stream?"

In today's market, delight and meaning are on the highest rungs of the value-stream ladder. One fast path to more currency is to ask yourself how you can exchange more delight and meaning in the marketplace, whether you're pitching your value to an employer or pitching a new product to the right prospect. As Jim Rohn says, "To have more, you simply have to become more. Don't wish for less problems, wish for more skills."[13] As you get better at this, your value generates currency. You become a master of financial fluency.

Because the money-value equation is an evolving current, what and even how you exchange value is a moving target. The marketplace rewards both adaptability and stability. One of my favorite questions I ask myself is, "Who do I need to become next to exchange more value in the marketplace?" I might need to become someone who looks for opportunities to be helpful to others. To brainstorm, write a list of ways you could respond to needs you see around you. This tunes your mind into generating opportunities. If you do this daily, you'll come up with something worth testing in your next season's or next year's milestones.

Metrics matter with currency. For example, ask yourself what number, what amount, of currency you want to generate this year. Then, reframe that in terms of value. How much value do you want to generate this year? This can help with the ideation process. Then, the process is what you already know: look at the critical issues, run small experiments, receive instant feedback, and look to add more value.

Perhaps you could directly fulfill some of the needs you see, given your time or expertise. Other needs might be opportunities to coordinate. For example, if your neighborhood needs dog walkers, and you're good at project coordinating, you could hire a part-time dog walker and manage a side business. You're not just generating revenue for yourself—you've added value to your neighbors and neighborhood (healthier dogs!), while also employing someone. (For more on adding value, I recommend *Company of One*, by Paul Jarvis, for both traditional employees and the self-employed.)

Next, notice what your three-year vision reveals about your desires. If your vision includes receiving more currency, how are you exploring how you will offer more value? As Csikszentmihalyi says, find where your skills meet peoples' challenges in the ever-changing marketplace, whether you are self-employed or part of an organization. Also, if you want to earn and invest more, notice how your favorite financially flush people follow their desire, trust their process, and continually add more value.

Whether you are part of a team or working on your own, you can provide unique value to your organization more than ever before. How do you choose which opportunities will add the most value by engaging your strengths to leverage them? Return to the Impact-Effort Grid to find the green tongue!

As we master water element, we become less afraid of gravity, of depth, of challenges. We start to understand difficulties as catalysts for flow and future expansion. When we swim in our internal waters, when we enter our own underworld, when we plumb our own depths, we accept the superpowers of water element. Accepting water, we say yes to self-compassion, to easeful effort, to growth, to increasing value, and to a life blessed with fluidity.

On this planet, life forms evolve from simplicity into complexity because of the presence of water. Water nourishes growth and creates the conditions to flourish in life. Mastering water helps us unlock flow, which brings with it the deepest satisfaction, where we are fully engaged, awake, and adding the most value with our unique abilities. Water reminds us to persist through surrender, to soften our edges, to heal, and to reveal through reflection. Water slows our pace by requiring patience, recalibration, and course correction, which eventually accelerate our growth and ability to reach our three-year vision. Like air, water encourages us to adapt ourselves to the changing circumstances, to evolve our identity to become what the situation requires, transforming a breakdown into our next breakthrough.

Space, air, and fire elements defy gravity and keep you above the surface of the earth in the field of growth. Earth forever reminds you to root into your body rhythms. Water brings gravity, reflection, smarter navigation. All five elements are forever present in each moment. Choosing to acknowledge the wisdom of our ancestors, to summon your abilities and intuition with the elements, leads you to mastery of you. You've made it through all five elements, and your power and prowess with the elements will continue to expand and deepen with iterations. Congratulations.

MASTER OF WATER (INTEGRITY AND FLOW)

○ When doubt and difficulty with your milestones arise, you reflect on your critical issues.

○ You seek to understand the underworld of your dharma and find parts of yourself that need to be integrated or evolved.

○ When challenges arise, you nourish yourself with healing waters and breath-body practices.

○ You use the Impact-Effort Grid to find the way to realign to your ambitions.

○ You fine-tune your skill-challenge balance to access the experience of flow.

○ You generate opportunities to add more value or exchange more value in your life.

○ You develop your depth and integrity to bolster your growth.

CONCLUSION:
WHO ARE YOU BECOMING?

Congratulations! You've been through a tour of *Master of You*. The actions you've taken and the exercises you've completed are now part of your lessons learned. You might start to see the elements at play in all aspects of your life. You've accessed the wisdom of Ayurveda and yoga through innovative life-skill building. You have a holistic operating system to manifest your ambitions on your own schedule, building a deep resilience in your body. Like all cycles, ends become beginnings. What you passed over or missed in this round is ready for your next round. You can use this system iteratively in a seasonal rhythm, continuously cycling into your next level of growth. In future iterations, you might focus on an element chapter a month. Eventually, cycling through the elements becomes natural.

If you've arrived at the end knowing you need to go back, to gain the powers of a certain element, I too have been there. At times in the long process of developing the Master of You global online course and community and writing this book, I wandered from an element or two. I skipped practices and exercises and blew off alignment meetings for months at a time. When I've procrastinated with fire's seasonal milestones and action plan or air's innovative calendar, I find stress mounting in my mind—like a tidal wave. With practice, I've come to know that feeling is part of the process, indicating it's time for action. Then the exercises are right there and take less time than expected because of past practice. You might find you've hit pause on one element while another element edged forward. The elements themselves will pull you back, like rain falling to the earth, into better alignment with your life, and you might notice the desire to modify the practices to suit your unique situation. For example, in doing the fire element exercises, I switched my team and family from quarterly planning cycles to triannual planning cycles. We spend less time planning and have an extra month to implement. If you keep returning to the system, you will find that breakthroughs and visions come into reality faster.

The Master of You system is now within you. In this concluding chapter, you'll see the progress you've made activating the elements into internal powers. I'll share one last practice—a personal favorite—that has helped me align to a continually expanding dharma. You'll also finish this book knowing which element(s) you need to focus on during your next iteration. With each pass through the system, the elements become you, and your intuition becomes stronger by activating their powers.

Pause for a quick assessment:

In which element(s) have you made big progress?

And which element(s) want(s) your attention right now?

You began this journey by reengineering your space to align with who you want to become next. If you are like many who have worked through this system, you likely found that starting outside of yourself, by mastering your space, shifted your ability to sense your deeper dreams with clarity. Then, you moved on to your inner space, descending from sky to earth, to your body, and optimized its rhythms and resilience with nourishment, movement, and sleep. With your intuitive trust gaining strength, you fired up your mental powers to envision your life's next chapter. Fire generated light, provoking insight to generate a better plan by clarifying your three-year vision, one-year milestones, and seasonal milestones. To pursue your vision, you worked to gain the power over time with air element. You morphed your calendar to meet your milestones, putting your strategy to the test of aligned action in real time. In putting your plan into action, you likely uncovered parts of yourself that needed to be developed to make your dreams come true. Growth requires integrity, so through your efforts, water might have swept you into your shadows, below the surface, and churned pressing critical issues into the light of day. With humility and compassion, you became a more integrated, more capable human through the process. In activating water element, you discovered the compelling reasons behind your dharma. Activating water often leads to adjusting your milestones to be truer to who you are right now, your authentic next purpose.

My hope and firm experience is that through this tour through the elements, *your* elements, you continually discover the next level of purpose, flow, delight, and meaning in your life . . . and are a boon to others.

GROUND YOUR EXPANSION

Your evolutionary journey is the path of being in the deepest joy, a state of en-joy-ment. This state comes from attentive, aligned effort. The yogis call this joy *ananda*, or awake to the field of bliss, which happens with more power in all five bodies: spiritual, physical, breath, mind, and intuitive. As you've been developing the elements, you've been developing these five koshas, or bodies. Space aligns to spirit, earth aligns to the body, fire aligns to the mind, air aligns to intuition, and water aligns to breath.

In activating your elements and your bodies, you are doing the intense work of tapas—the heat generated from burning off impurities—which results in evolutionary actions. Through the high-vibration friction of pulsing between depth and growth, you generate insight and light—you become more en-light-ened. Your future is even brighter. And as a result, you can continually access heartfelt meaning and mind-blowing fulfillment: this is ananda, or bliss. You will notice with greater sensitivity the relationship between cause and effect—the law of karma. As you absorb even more subtle lessons learned, you cultivate increased sensitivity, like enhanced radar, on your evolutionary journey. Yet, greater sensitivity also means that you have a shorter leash with heeding the call of your intuition and not repeating the same lessons learned. When honored, this becomes a positive feedback loop that compounds into exponential growth. As you become even more of a master of you, you will experience bigger wins—breakthroughs on the way to your ambitions—so you want to ground your breakthroughs physically and energetically through your body. Increasing your tolerance for positivity, for things to go right in a bigger way, is a learned skill.

Gay Hendricks explains this phenomenon in *The Big Leap*: "Each of us has an inner thermostat setting that determines how much love, success, and creativity we allow ourselves to enjoy. When we exceed our inner thermostat setting, we will often do something to sabotage ourselves, causing us to drop back into the old, familiar zone where we feel secure."[1] Hendricks labels this unconscious self-sabotage the "Upper Limit Problem," which happens as you attempt to evolve beyond the familiar, or the limited, mind. As humans, we have self-reflective awareness that enables us to see our own limited thinking and evolve beyond it.

Let's delve into beliefs that defy the normal. One expanded belief is that your essential and elemental nature is the same as the essential and elemental nature of the universe. The universe is bigger and expands faster than the speed of light. If we follow this logic, your potential as part of the cosmos is expanding beyond what you might have previously imagined. According to Strategic Coach founder Dan Sullivan, when two people come together who are living in their "unique ability," they can go 100 times bigger in their goals.[2] This experience of Sullivan's comes from 50/50 joint ventures he has coached organizations through and done himself. The idea of the compound effect is not to limit yourself based on your past experience, and Hendricks has two antidotes.

His first solution to the Upper Limit Problem is a mantra that calibrates the mind to expansion: "I expand in abundance, success, and love every day, as I inspire those around me to do the same."[3] Half of the brilliance of this mantra is the noncompetitive, sharing nature of true prosperity. The universal imperative is that we grow together, that what is good for me is also good for you and vice versa. Exponential growth happens when we help each other, and the synergy can amplify. As Stephen Covey explains in *The 3rd Alternative: Solving Life's Most Difficult Problems*, "Synergy is what happens when one plus one equals ten or a hundred or even a thousand! It's the profound result when two or more respectful human beings determine to go beyond their preconceived ideas to meet a great challenge."[4] Experiencing exponential growth and being awake to synergy is a spiritual practice, and like any practice, it requires practice to master.

Hendricks's second practice is to gradually and consistently expand your tolerance for the natural good feelings that come with growth by savoring them as they arise. Although this sounds obvious, most people find that until they make this part of their mindfulness practice, they don't do it. If you pause to practice it a few times daily, you'll see your ability to feel good expand.

The next exercise is a body-mind practice that expands and roots the good feeling both physically and energetically into the body. I've found that this practice is essential for consistently shattering glass ceilings in the multiple arenas of modern life. You will steer your attention into your body so that your cells absorb the sensations of more abundance, success, love, or any other benefits of your previous breakthrough. After you do an alignment meeting or hit one of your seasonal milestones, do this practice.

This practice calibrates your cells for growth. You want to overcome any tendencies toward limitations or setbacks in your energy body. If you don't recalibrate expansion after a breakthrough, you reinforce your own limitations. You want to train yourself to consistently become a better, brighter, and more skillful version of yourself. This is a fast way to grow beyond previous unconscious limits. Incorporate this quick, invaluable practice in small, yet noticeable, grace-filled moments during the day or before sleep.

Recalibrating Practice
(Listen to the recording at masterofyou.us/workbook.)

1. Stand with your feet more than hip-width apart, with a slight bend in your knees, to relax your weight into your feet.

2. Open your chest with slower, fuller breathing, and let your arms hang with palms open. As you exhale, relax.

3. Notice and feel into the sensations in your body of feeling good, of expanding into what is working in your life. Allow your body to absorb, receive, and digest this experience. You might feel your body relax and expand. Notice or imagine that your cells are now operating at a higher frequency—a frequency that can hold more light. Remind yourself of the word *enlightened*—being in light.

4. Remember your connection to the expanding universe and expand your upper limit for all that is positive. Embody this as your "new normal." You are alchemizing the next level of you, recalibrating your awareness. Feel this frequency, the sensations of feeling stronger positive vibrations all the way through your legs and feet. You are becoming "grounded" in the vibrational "new normal" of your body.

Do this recalibration exercise daily, especially when doing small tests and failing fast and when positive results start rolling in on your three-year vision. Then, notice what ideas, thoughts, and workflows happen as a result. This practice builds your momentum with success, and that success compounds. As you experience the powers of the elements—both in big *and* small ways—pause and recalibrate. Build this habit to feel and familiarize your cells with the evolving vibration of who you are becoming. ■

LEADER OF US

In working with the elements within you, you are mastering your direction, your life of meaning, your legacy. Your awareness encompasses both being and becoming, content with who you are right now and who you are becoming in your next identity. The elements are energies within and outside of you, and they are also your inspiration and your building blocks for creation. You are becoming the master of you.

Please humor one last word of advice: We humans often misinterpret the issues that arise on our journey to our deeper dreams as bad, so we shrink from the dreams. When you can see this contraction, your limitations, you can initiate the next phase of the cycle—your opportunity, your expansion. This is how spanda works. As Susan B. Anthony famously said, "Cautious, careful people, always casting about to preserve their reputations, can never effect a reform."[5] So, keep acquiring your powers with the elements to become even more rooted, experimental, strategic, and curious, and then be bold about what you are able to do and become next (see Figure C1).

BIGGER DHARMA AND IDENTITY EVOLUTION SPIRAL

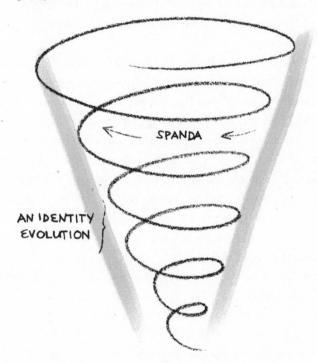

THE BEGINNING: FOLLOWING DEEPER DESIRES INTO ALIGNED ACTION

Figure C1 Stepping into a bigger dharma grows your identity into a more powerful and expansive version of yourself.

Continue to work with the elements, and explore and experience their more subtle energies. Soon, you'll embrace all of the weather of the elements without preference: the rain of water, the heat of fire, the wind of air. Some people like to work through the five elements and the Master of You exercises annually, others join my global online course for guidance and community, and some start book clubs of their own (see more information about this under Book Club Ideas later in the book). Others revisit it during transitions, difficult periods, and times of growth.

With self-mastery comes leadership. As you become skillful and gain the core competencies of the elements, people will notice and become inspired. Through you, people can sense and access their own creative potential. Your discipline to the body rhythms and your dedication to your potential, your dharma, your vision, and your achievements are noticeable and noticed.

As you become masterful with the elements, you'll likely attract or be drawn to people awake to their creative power who have built inner resilience and who have accessed the same elemental, universal truths you have. You'll be increasingly drawn to collaborate with people rooted in their powers and reaching to become more, sensing themselves and the cosmos. New, more evolved possibilities and collaborations arise. You are waking up to another level of impact, or dharma, of your human capacity. You might even sense a collaborative spirit, a collective potentiality. You are entering the dynamic of collective leadership, in which you can access new dimensions of collaboration and innovation.

Activated by the elements, you'll notice you are being pulled or called to lead. People sense your rooted, aligned power and are attracted to you. Master of You evolves into Leader of Us. Where you lead us is part of your dharma unfolding, powered by the elements, awake and intuitively attracted to aligned, unique visions and synergistic potentials. Holistic leaders are discovering and experimenting with new ground rules, insights, and exercises that activate collective leadership. How are you being called to lead? Notice that. Like Susan B. Anthony leading the reform, your community—however grand or small—is calling on you to be and to lead the evolution. By reading this book and doing the work to be self-empowered by the elements, you are part of this collective evolution. You are leading yourself. As a leader, you honor your dharma—your purpose—even as it expands, requiring you to evolve on your path of becoming. You lead us.

You are the cosmos.
You are the cosmos that created you.
You create via the five elements, out of possibility, toward excellence.
You are the magic and the myth.
You are the hero and the journey.
And yet.
You are ordinary.
You lead an ordinary life, like the rest of us.
And yet.
You are extraordinary.
Even in the hustle bustle of today, you remember. You and the creator are one, the same. The five elements are your powers to shape yourself and your cosmos. You design you for your next chapter of dharma.
You hear opportunity knocking.
You become a beacon for those around you to unearth their deeper dreams, fire up their ambitions, discover their inner rhythm, free their time, unleash their flow. In your experiments, you are an inspiration to those around you of being and becoming, like the cosmos, both at ease and ambitious. You wield the elements and grow in ever-increasing integrity and capacity.
You shape your world. You choose your next identity and shape-shift. You are a master of being and belonging and becoming—a master of you.
Activated with the wisdom of the elements, you lead us.

ACKNOWLEDGMENTS

It takes a village for me to raise a book. Thank you to the original members of Awake Living—the course and community behind Master of You—for believing in the process and experimenting with me to make it into the system it is today, especially Dana Skoglund and Rachel Peters. To the members of Body Thrive for living the habits and orienting themselves toward thrive. Thanks to the Yogahealer.com Yoga Health Coaches for doing the good work of guiding your people to thrive in their bodies and their lives. To Gretel for kicking the butt of this manuscript into a book. For Jaime at Sounds True for seeing the potential of *Master of You* to be an innovative expression of Ayurveda.

And of course, to Winston and Indy for not giving me too much flack for packing the laptop into the boat, into the camper, and on every plane and automobile trip . . . and for making sure I closed it to enjoy our precious life together along the way. And to Mom for giving me your big heart and always knowing I could do it, and Dad for giving me your sharp mind and respecting what it takes to write a good book and grow a good company.

NOTES

INTRODUCTION WHO COULD YOU BECOME NEXT?

1. Bob Anderson and William Adams, *Mastering Leadership: An Integrated Framework for Breakthrough Performance and Extraordinary Business Results* (Hoboken, NJ: Wiley, 2015).

2. Elaine Pofeldt, "How More Women Can Break the $1 Million Mark," *Forbes*, September 28, 2018, forbes.com/sites/elainepofeldt/2018/09/28/how-more-women-can-break-the-1-million-mark/#54b858087df1.

CHAPTER 1 UNEARTH YOUR DEEPER DREAM TO AWAKEN YOUR AMBITION

1. Barrett C. Brown, "Overview of Developmental Stages of Consciousness," Integral Without Borders, April 3, 2006, integralwithoutborders.net/sites/default/files/resources/Overview%20of%20Developmental%20Levels.pdf.

2. Robert Aitken, "The Bodhisattva Vows," *Tricycle* (Summer 1992), tricycle.org/magazine/bodhisattva-vows/.

3. Thomas Merton, *No Man Is an Island* (New York: Mariner, 2002), 133.

4. Stephen Cope, *The Great Work of Your Life* (New York: Random House, 2015), xxi.

5. Christopher Bergland, "How Do Neuroplasticity and Neurogenesis Rewire Your Brain?" *Psychology Today*, February 6, 2017, psychologytoday.com/us/blog/the-athletes-way/201702/how-do-neuroplasticity-and-neurogenesis-rewire-your-brain.

6. Marshall Goldsmith and Mark Reiter, *Triggers: Creating Behavior That Lasts—Becoming the Person You Want to Be* (New York: Crown, 2015), xix.

7. Joseph Campbell, *The Hero with a Thousand Faces* (Novato, CA: New World Library, 2008), 49.

CHAPTER 2   INNOVATING WITH THE FIVE PRIMORDIAL ELEMENTS

1. Other traditions, such as Chinese medicine, use different elements with similar concepts: wood, fire, earth, metal, water.

2. Vasant Lad, *Textbook of Ayurveda*, vol. 1 (Albuquerque, NM: Ayurvedic Press, 2002), 26.

3. Vasant Lad, "The Five Elements and Ayurvedic Medicine," Ayurveda College, ayurvedacollege.com/book/export/html/560.

4. "Auto Immune Disease Statistics," American Autoimmune Related Disease Association, aarda.org/news-information/statistics/; "Women & Autoimmunity," American Autoimmune Related Disease Association, aarda.org/who-we-help/patients/women-and-autoimmunity/.

5. Allie Johnson, "Poll: No End in Sight for 2 out of 3 US Adults with Debt," January 9, 2019, creditcards.com/credit-card-news/debt-free-living-poll.php.

6. US Geological Survey, "The Water in You: Water in the Human Body," usgs.gov/special-topic/water-science-school/science/water-you-water-and-human-body?qt-science_center_objects=0#qt-science_center_objects.

7. Anderson and Adams, *Mastering Leadership*, xxvi.

8. James Clear, *Atomic Habits: An Easy and Proven Way to Build Good Habits and Break Bad Ones* (New York: Avery, 2018), 28.

9. Goldsmith and Reiter, *Triggers*.

10. Strategic Coach, now.strategiccoach.com/howtogetothetop.

CHAPTER 3   MASTER OF YOU ETHOS

1. George Forsythe, Karen Kuhla, and Daniel Rice, "Understanding the Challenges of a VUCA Environment," Chief Executive, May 15, 2018, chiefexecutive.net/understanding-vuca-environment/.

2. Jane McGonigal, *SuperBetter: The Power of Living Gamefully* (New York: Penguin, 2015).

3. "Don't Rest after Victory, Failure Just an Attempt at Learning: A. P. J. Abdul Kalam," *Economic Times*, July 28, 2015, economictimes.indiatimes.com/news/politics-and-nation/dont-rest-after-victory-failure-just-an-attempt-at-learning-a-p-j-abdul-kalam/articleshow/48249644.cms.

4. Carol S. Dweck, *Mindset: The New Psychology of Success* (New York: Random House, 2006).

5. Kristen Wheeler, "Learn How Your Native Genius Works," nativegenius.com/native-genius-faqs/.

6. Susan Gunelius, "The Shift from CONsumers to PROsumers," *Forbes*, July 3, 2010, forbes.com/sites/work-in-progress/2010/07/03/the-shift-from-consumers-to-prosumers/#2a2c459a33df.

7. Clear, *Atomic Habits*, 38.

CHAPTER 4 SPACE: MASTER OF HOME

1. Lad, *Textbook of Ayurveda*, vol. 1, 13.

2. Benjamin Hardy, *Willpower Doesn't Work: Discover the Hidden Keys to Success* (New York: Hachette, 2018), Kindle Edition, 632–634.

3. Ralph Bergstresser, "Comments from the Inventor of Purple Harmony Plates," bibliotecapleyades.net/ciencia/esp_ciencia_universalenergy02.htm.

4. Marie Kondo, *The Life-Changing Magic of Tidying Up: The Japanese Art of Decluttering and Organizing* (Berkeley, CA: Ten Speed Press, 2014).

5. Hardy, *Willpower Doesn't Work*, 510.

6. Michael Stone, "A Deeper Materialism," October 13, 2013, TEDxToronto presentation, michaelstoneteaching.com/2013/10/13/a-deeper-materialism-michael-stone-at-tedxtoronto/.

7. Stone, "Deeper Materialism."

8. "Resonance," Physics Classroom, physicsclassroom.com/class/sound/Lesson-5/Resonance.

9. "Health Risks of a Sedentary Lifestyle," LifeSpan Fitness, April 13, 2017, lifespanfitness.com/workplace/resources/articles/health-risks-of-a-sedentary-lifestyle.

10. Charles Duhigg, *The Power of Habit: Why We Do What We Do in Life and Business* (New York: Doubleday, 2012).

CHAPTER 5 EARTH: MASTER OF BODY

1. National Institute of General Medical Sciences, "Circadian Rhythms," nigms.nih.gov/education/pages/factsheet_circadianrhythms.aspx.

2. Robert Svoboda, *Prakriti: Your Ayurvedic Constitution* (Twin Lakes, WI: Lotus Press, 1988), 123.

3. Jorge Alejandro Alegría-Torres, Andrea Baccarelli, and Valentina Bollati, "Epigenetics and Lifestyle," *Epigenomics* 3, no. 3 (2011): 267–277.

4. Michael F. Picco, "Digestion: How Long Does It Take?" Mayo Clinic, September 27, 2018, mayoclinic.org/digestive-system/expert-answers/faq-20058340.

5. Vasant Lad, *Textbook of Ayurveda*, vol. 2: A Complete Guide to Clinical Assessment (Albuquerque NM: Ayurvedic Press, 2006), 190, 199–202.

6. John Douillard, "Blood Sugar," LifeSpa, lifespa.com/ayurvedic-treatment-health-topics/blood-sugar/.

7. Valter D. Longo and Satchidananda Panda, "Fasting, Circadian Rhythms, and Time Restricted Feeding," *Cell Metabolism* 23, no. 6 (June 14, 2016): 1048–1059, ncbi.nlm.nih.gov/pmc/articles/PMC5388543/.

8. Marjet J. M. Munsters and Wim H. M. Saris, "Effects of Meal Frequency on Metabolic Profiles and Substrate Partitioning in Lean Healthy Males," *PLOS One* 7, no. 6 (June 13, 2012): ncbi.nlm.nih.gov/pmc/articles/PMC5388543/; John Douillard, "The Dangers of Frequent Eating," LifeSpa, lifespa.com/dangers-of-frequent-eating/.

9. Hana Kahleova et al., "Eating Two Larger Meals a Day (Breakfast and Lunch) Is More Effective Than Six Smaller Meals in a Reduced-Energy Regimen for Patients with Type 2 Diabetes: A Randomized Crossover Study," *Diabetologia* 57, no. 8 (May 18, 2014): 1552–1560, ncbi.nlm.nih.gov/pmc/articles/PMC4079942/.

10. Lilli Link, "Are You Inflamed? Five Signs to Look Out For," Parsley Health Articles, parsleyhealth.com/blog/5-signs-chronic-inflammation/.

11. C. Gupta and D. Prakash, "Phytonutrients as Therapeutic Agents," *Journal of Complementary Integrative Medicine* 11, no. 3 (September 11, 2014): 151–169, ncbi.nlm.nih.gov/pubmed/25051278.

12. Jean L. Wiecha et al., "Household Television Access: Associations with Screen Time, Reading, and Homework among Youth," *Ambulatory Pediatrics* 1, no. 5 (September–October 2001): 244–251, sciencedirect.com/science/article/pii/S1530156705600548?via%3Dihub.

13. "Health Risks of an Inactive Lifestyle," *Medline Plus*, sciencedirect. com/science/article/pii/S1530156705600548?via%3Dihub.

14. Daniela Schmid and Graham Colditz, "Sedentary Behavior Increases the Risk of Certain Cancers," *JNCI: Journal of the National Cancer Institute* 106, no. 7 (July 2014), academic.oup.com/jnci/ article/106/7/dju206/1010488.

15. Roy J. Shephard and Robin Futcher, "Physical Activity and Cancer: How May Protection Be Maximized?" *Critical Reviews on Oncogenesis* 8, nos. 2–3 (1997): 219–272, dl.begellhouse.com/journals/439f422d 0783386a,703283381dd19c5b,62bbd564563e4435.html.

16. Joseph A. Knight, "Physical Inactivity: Associated Diseases and Disorders," *Annals of Clinical and Laboratory Science* 42, no. 3 (Summer 2012): 320–337, annclinlabsci.org/content/42/3/320.full.

17. Alisa Hrustic, "Seven Surprising Ways You Wreck Your Body When You Don't Get Off Your Butt," *Men's Health*, March 1, 2017, menshealth.com/health/g19541989/ effects-of-sedentary-lifestyle/?slide=1.

18. US Department of Health and Human Services, *Your Guide to Healthy Sleep*, National Institutes of Health Publication No. 11-5271, November 2005, nhlbi.nih.gov/files/docs/public/sleep/healthy_sleep. pdf.

19. Cate Stillman, *Body Thrive* (Boulder, CO: Sounds True, 2019).

20. Allison Aubrey, "Drivers Beware: Crash Rate Hikes with Every Hour of Lost Sleep," *All Things Considered*, National Public Radio, December 6, 2016, npr.org/ sections/health-shots/2016/12/06/504448639/ drivers-beware-crash-rate-spikes-with-every-hour-of-lost-sleep.

21. Eve Van Cauter et al., "The Impact of Sleep Deprivation on Hormones and Metabolism," Medscape (2005), medscape.org/ viewarticle/502825.

22. Stephen Watson and Kristeen Cherney, "The Effects of Sleep Deprivation on the Body," Healthline, April 19, 2019, healthline. com/health/sleep-deprivation/effects-on-body#1.

23. Andrew Goliszek, "The Stress-Sex Connection," *Psychology Today*, December 22, 2014, psychologytoday.com/us/blog/how- the-mind-heals-the-body/201412/the-stress-sex-connection; K. Uvnas-Modberg and M. Petersson, "Oxytocin: A Mediator of

Anti-Stress, Well-Being, Social Interaction, Growth, and Healing, *Zeitschrift für Psychosomatische Medizin und Psychotherapie* 51, no. 1 (2005): 57–80.

CHAPTER 6   FIRE: MASTER OF AMBITION

1. Jordan B. Peterson, *12 Rules for Life: An Antidote to Chaos* (Toronto: Random House), 282.

2. Peterson, *12 Rules for Life*, 282.

3. Jim Collins and Jerry Porras, *Built to Last: Successful Habits of Visionary Companies* (New York: Harper Collins, 2011).

4. Paul Jarvis, *Company of One: Why Staying Small Is the Next Big Thing for Business* (New York: Houghton Mifflin Harcourt, 2019).

5. Clarissa Pinkola Estés, *Women Who Run with the Wolves: Myths and Stories of the Wild Woman Archetype* (New York: Ballantine, 1996).

6. Tytus Michalski, "Five Questions with Dave Gray: Liminal Thinking, Doom Loops, Attention, Beliefs, Filter Bubbles, and More," *Medium*, February 1, 2017.

7. Quote Investigator, quoteinvestigator.com/2014/03/29/sharp-axe/.

8. Brian P. Moran and Michael Lennington, *The 12 Week Year: Get More Done in 12 Weeks Than Others Get Done in 12 Months* (Hoboken, NJ: Wiley, 2013).

9. Svoboda, *Prakriti*, 127.

10. Svoboda, *Prakriti*, 126.

11. "J. P. Morgan Biography," IMDB, imdb.com/name/nm2393073/bio.

12. Tyler Norton, Elite Forum workshops, Phoenix, Arizona, 2017 and 2018.

13. Haruki Murakami, "Cream," *The New Yorker*, January 29, 2019, 65.

CHAPTER 7   AIR: MASTER OF TIME

1. Nola Taylor Redd, "How Fast Does Light Travel?" *Space*, March 7, 2018, space.com/15830-light-speed.html.

2. Redd, "How Fast Does Light Travel?"

3. Syed Muhammad Sajjad Kabir, "Stress and Time Management," researchgate.net/publication/325546110_STRESS_AND_TIME_MANAGEMENT.

4. American Psychological Association, "APA Survey Raises Concern about Health Impact of Stress on Children and Families," November 9, 2010, apa.org/news/press/releases/2010/11/stress-in-america.

5. Mayo Clinic, "Chronic Stress Puts Your Health at Risk," mayoclinic. org/healthy-lifestyle/stress-management/in-depth/stress/ art-20046037.

6. Ian LeSueur, "Subjective Time and Mindfulness," *Keep*, January 1, 2014, thekeep.eiu.edu/cgi/viewcontent.cgi?referer= google.com/&htt psredir=1&article=2265&context=theses.

7. Stephen Sturgess, *The Yoga Book: A Practical and Spiritual Guide to Self-Realization* (London: Watkins, 2015).

8. R. L. Siegel, K. D. Miller, and A. Jemal, "Cancer Statistics, 2015," *Cancer Journal for Clinicians* 65, no. 1 (January–February 2015): 5–29, ncbi.nlm.nih.gov/pubmed/25559415l; Marc A. Russo, Danielle M. Santarelli, and Dean O'Rourke, "The Physiological Effects of Slow Breathing in the Healthy Human," *Breathe* 13, no. 4 (December 2017): 298–309, ncbi.nlm.nih.gov/pmc/articles/ PMC5709795/.

9. Waleed O. Twal, Amy E. Wahlquist, and Sundaravadivel Balasubramanian, "Yogic Breathing When Compared to Attention Control Reduces the Levels of Pro-Inflammatory Biomarkers in Salvia: A Pilot Randomized Controlled Trial," *BMC Complementary and Alternative Medicine*, August 18, 2016, bmccomplementalternmed.biomedcentral.com/articles/10.1186/ s12906-016-1286-7.

10. Russo, Santarelli, and O'Rourke, "The Physiological Effects of Slow Breathing in the Healthy Human."

11. Peterson, *12 Rules for Life*, 283.

12. Peterson, *12 Rules for Life*, 283.

13. Dan Sullivan, "How to Stay on Top of Your Entrepreneurial Game," resources.strategiccoach.com/the-multiplier-mindset-blog/ how-to-stay-at-the-top-of-your-entrepreneurial-game-2.

14. Moran and Lennington, *The 12 Week Year*.

15. Dan Schawbel, "Jocko Willink: The Relationship Between Discipline and Freedom," *Forbes*, October 17, 2017, forbes.com/sites/ danschawbel/2017/10/17/jocko-willink-the-relationship-between- discipline-and-freedom/#3a1840516df8.

16. Clear, *Atomic Habits*, 19.

17. Clear, *Atomic Habits*, 19.

CHAPTER 8 WATER: MASTER OF INTEGRITY AND FLOW

1. John Heider, *The Tao of Leadership: Lao Tzu's* Tao Te Ching *Adapted for a New Age* (Atlanta: Green Dragon, 2005), 78.

2. Pacifica Graduate Institute, "What Is Depth Psychology?" pacifica. edu/about-pacifica/what-is-depth-psychology/.

3. Richard Graves, *Meditations of the Emperor Marcus Aurelius Antoninus: A New Translation from the Greek Original* (Farmington Hills, MI: Gale, 2010), 20.

4. C. G. Jung, *The Collected Works of Carl Jung*, vol. 9 (part 2): *Aion: Researches into the Phenomenology of the Self* (Princeton, NJ: Princeton University Press, 2014), chap. 5.

5. Jim Rohn quotes, youtube.com/watch?v=8yG7N9NrQ8c.

6. Christopher Bergland, "Self-Compassion, Growth Mindset, and Benefits of Failure," *Psychology Today*, January 30, 2017, psychologytoday.com/us/blog/the-athletes-way/201701/ self-compassion-growth-mindset-and-the-benefits-failure.

7. Lad, *Textbook of Ayurveda*, vol. 1, 137.

8. "The Science Behind the Wim Hof Method," wimhofmethod.com/ science.

9. "The Science Behind the Wim Hof Method," wimhofmethod.com/ science.

10. James Altucher, *Choose Yourself! Be Happy, Make Millions, Live the Dream* (New York: Author, 2013).

11. Mihaly Csikszentmihalyi. "Introduction," in *Optimal Experience: Psychological Studies of Flow in Consciousness* (Cambridge, UK: Cambridge University Press, 1998).

12. Mihaly Csikszentmihalyi, *Flow: The Psychology of Optimal Experience* (New York: HarperCollins, 1991).

13. Jim Rohn quotes, youtube.com/watch?v=8yG7N9NrQ8c.

CONCLUSION WHO ARE YOU BECOMING?

1. Gay Hendricks, *The Big Leap: Conquer Your Hidden Fear and Take Life to the Next Level* (New York: HarperCollins, 2010), 20.

2. Dan Sullivan, "Why Stop at 10x? How Collaboration Can Lead to 100x Growth," July 26, 2018, strategicpodcasts.com/podcast/inside-strategic-coach/episode/why-stop-at-10x-how-collaboration-can-lead-to-100x-growth/.

3. Hendricks, *Big Leap*, 20.

4. Stephen Covey, *The 3rd Alternative: Solving Life's Most Difficult Problems* (New York: Free Press, 2012), 12.

5. Alma Lutz, *Susan B. Anthony: Rebel, Crusader, Humanitarian* (New York: Pantianos, 1959), 70.

GLOSSARY

Earth my body
Water my blood
Air my breath
Fire my spirit

—Native American prayer

AGNI: Fire; in Ayurveda meaning digestive fire and the power of cells to digest and transform; related to sense of vision, third chakra, ambition

AKASHA: Space, related to sense of hearing, fifth chakra, spiritual evolution

AKRAMA: Lack of intelligent sequencing that can break down order into disharmony and confusion

AMA: Poorly undigested food that becomes toxic to the body

ANANDA: The natural state of intrinsic ease and joy, arising from our inner nature

APANA: The downward flow of energy in the body, which causes the exhale, the release of urine and feces, menses, and childbirth

APAS: Water, related to sense of taste, second chakra, healing

AYURVEDA: The art and science of understanding life, healing, and thriving; *Ayur* = life, *Veda* = knowledge

DHARMA: Traditionally refers to duty and sacrifice, to uphold virtue, and to good works; one of the four aims of life. The modern meaning is to uphold your unique purpose as it transforms through the stages of your life.

DOSHAS: The three energies that create the constitution of everything living—anabolism (kapha), metabolism (pitta), and catabolism (vata).

DUKKHA: Dirty space; the suffering that arises from unclarified space element.

ISHVARA PRANIDHANA: Offering personal purpose to a greater good; allowing the supreme, the highest, source energy to power one's efforts and guide one's intuition

KAIZEN: The philosophy of small, continuous improvement, arising from a Japanese business philosophy

KAPHA: To flourish by water. It's one of the triadic forces, or doshas (along with pitta and vata). Kapha generates cohesion or holding cells together, protection, and repair. Kaphas' qualities are heavy, slow, steady, solid, cold, soft, and oily.

KARMA: The law of cause and effect, and accumulation of past actions

KRAMA: Chronology, or a special sequence in time, used to create a desired effect

LILA: the play of the cosmos unfolding in freedom and creativity

MEDAS DHATU: The adipose tissue, the stable fuel source for the body; related to water element, kapha dosha, joint lubrication, and the psychological experiences of love, connection, and acceptance

PITTA: One of the triadic forces, or doshas (along with kapha and vata). Pitta controls digestion, metabolism, and energy production. The primary function of pitta is transformation. The qualities of pitta are hot, light, intense, penetrating, pungent, sharp, and acidic.

PRANA: The life-giving, intelligent force of the breath, which coordinates our cells, senses, and mind. It is the subtle energy of vata behind all mind-body functions and the catalyst for manifestation and evolution. When your prana is optimal, you become aware, flexible, adaptable, and growth oriented.

PRANAYAMA: A yogic conscious-breathing practice designed to optimize one's vital energy

PRITHVI: Earth, related to sense of smell, root chakra, established in the body

PURNA: Fullness or completeness

SADHANA: A practice or discipline that leads to an aligned life

SAMSKARAS: Recycled or stuck behavioral or thought patterns as a result of perpetuating tendencies in the subconscious mind

SHAKTI: The female principle of divine energy moving and manifesting the universe

SHIVAYA: The male principle of divine beneficence and auspiciousness—life is inherently good

SPANDA: The universal principle of vibration connected to the law of polarity—the pulsations between expansion and contraction with everything and everyone (unmesha and nimesha together are spanda)

STHIRA: Stillness that comes from awareness of being or mindfulness

SUKHA: Clean space; implies the ease that arises from aligned action

SVASTHA: Seated in the self, or self-aware and embodied—one of the conditions of health in Ayurveda

SVATANTRYA: Describes that our inner nature is completely free

TAPAS: The rub or heat generated by disciplined action; tapas renders light

TARPAKA KAPHA: The subdosha of kapha that enables memory retention and memory retrieval

TEJAS: Our inner radiance, derived from the subtle energy of fire and the positive essence of pitta dosha; tejas fires up our drive and aspirations to evolve

VAIRAGYA: Practice without attachment to results, or working a process for the sake of learning without clinging to the outcome

VATA: One of the triadic forces, or doshas (along with kapha and pitta). Vata governs movement in the body, including breath, circulation, digestion, elimination, and nervous system activity. It moves the other doshas. Its qualities are cold, light, dry, irregular, rough, moving, quick, and changeable.

VAYU: Air or wind; related to sense of touch, heart chakra, creativity, and spontaneity

VIVEKA: Discrimination, or the action or ability to distinguish or perceive differences. It is the power to differentiate between right and wrong, real and apparent, eternal and transient, better and worse.

YOGA: The art of yoking one's personal mind, body, and spirit to universal consciousness and planetary interconnectivity, awakening one's potential for the good of all

RESOURCES

ETHOS

Mindset by Carol Dweck
Liminal Thinking by Dave Gray
SuperBetter by Jane McGonigal
12 Rules of Life by Jordan Peterson
Strengths 2.0 by Tom Rath

SPACE ELEMENT

The Life-Changing Magic of Tidying Up by Marie Kondo
"A Deeper Materialism" TEDx Talk by Michael Stone
Willpower Doesn't Work by Benjamin Hardy

EARTH ELEMENT

Body Thrive by Cate Stillman
Sleep with Me podcast by Drew Ackerman
Balance Your Hormones, Balance Your Life by Claudia Welch
The Everyday Ayurveda Cookbook by Kate O'Donnell
Atomic Habits by James Clear

FIRE ELEMENT

Traction by Gene Wickman
Strategic Intuition by William Duggan
Creative Strategy: A Guide for Innovation by William Duggan
Company of One by Paul Jarvis

AIR ELEMENT

The 12 Week Year by Brian Moran and Michael Lennington
Multiplier Mindset podcast by Dan Sullivan
Zen to Done by Leo Babauta
"Inside the Mind of a Master Procrastinator" Ted Talk by Tim Urban
Compound Effect podcast by Darren Hardy

WATER ELEMENT

Descent to the Goddess: A Way of Initiation for Women by Sylvia Brinton Perera
The Heroine's Journey by Maureen Murdock
When God Was a Woman by Merlin Stone
The Chalice and the Blade by Riane Eisler
Jungian philosophy

AYURVEDA AND YOGA

Yoga Sutras by Patanjali
Prakriti by Robert Svoboda

INDEX

eating, 42, 87, 92, 93
   fasting and, 53, 99, 104
   rhythmic, 97, 99–104, 111, 114
efficiency, 8, 32, 34, 71, 100, 143, 146
   evolutionary, 11–14
ego, xvi
   surrendering, 163
elements. See five elements
emotions, 10, 38, 77, 81, 82, 107, 163,
      165, 166, 213
   breathing and, 95
   digesting, 95–96
   dynamic learning and, 13
   evolution of, 159
   mind and, 92, 95
   positive, 35, 50, 109
   processing, 78, 89, 102
   rebalancing, 172
   repressed, 99
   specific, 97
   stressed-out, 140
emptiness, 73, 95, 102, 104
energy, xvii, 38, 73, 95, 96, 100, 113,
      151, 174
   absorbing, 173
   best use of, 17
   downward, 91
   emotional, 166
   improving, ix, 57
   inner, 172
   life-force, 23, 24
   low, 103
   movement and, 96
   quick-start, 118
   rooting, 91
   stable, 35
   subtle, 188
   trusting, 60
   universal, 24, 45
enoughness, 18, 59
environment, xii, xiii, xiv, 72
   creating/controlling, 33
   designing, 86–87
   habitual, 121
   peak-performance, 88
   restructuring, 73, 86–88
   upgrading, 71
Estés, Clarissa Pinkola, 120
ethos, xvi, xxi, 28, 68, 69, 81, 89, 154
   collective, 81
   discussing, 67, 212

mastering, 42–43
personal, 34, 41, 42
resources for, 207
evolution, xvi, 10, 18–19
   collective, 64, 189
   cycles of, 60
   desire and, xvii
   emotional, 160
   identity, 5, 11, 52, 153, 167
   personal, 5, 6, 14, 28, 55, 147–51
   testing small/thinking big for, 54
   time and, 153
Evolutionaries (Hubbard), 17
exercise, xv, xvi, 44, 107, 110, 112,
      119, 124, 181–82
   contemplation, 122
   doing, 108, 109, 211
exhaling, 28, 95, 102, 103, 142, 143,
      156, 173, 185
expansion, x, xix, 137, 143, 166, 187
   contraction and, x
   grounding, 183–85
   space element and, 139
experience, x, 11, 39, 71, 84, 118, 130, 186
   dharma and, 7
   lived, 77
   transforming, 10
experimentation, 56, 103–4, 149
   continual, 55, 113

failing fast, 43, 54–56
failure, 163
   reframing, 55
   success and, 152
Farhi, Donna, 103
fasting, 100, 101, 103, 113, 114
   eating and, 53, 99, 104
fat, 114
   fabulous, 105
   flipping, 100–103
   nutrient-dense, 106
fat metabolism, 101, 103, 114
feedback, 101, 113, 159, 177
   instant, 58
   learning, 55
   negative, 16
   positive, 183
feeling, 25, 74, 96, 186
   good, 185
   negative, 93

habits, xvii, 34, 47, 71, 81, 84, 86, 89,
    96, 154
  aligned, 93
  arrhythmic, 94
  automating, xix, 49
  bad, 100, 152
  body, 23, 124
  culture and, 41, 98 (fig.)
  daily, xiv, 93, 94
  developing, 41, 51, 94, 155, 176
  flow, 176
  goals and, 155
  good, 98, 152, 156
  improving/refining, 23, 35, 87
  mental/emotional, 19
  messaging and, 87
  past/presence and, 94
  space and, 72–79, 88
  triggers and, 87
Hardy, Benjamin, 72, 81
headaches, xi, 103, 106, 128, 141
healing, 159, 162
  autoimmune, 171
  water element and, 37
health, xi, xii, xiv, 93, 112
  resilience and, 93
  transformation of, xvi
health issues, xiii, 99, 106
  healing, xiv
  reducing, 107
Hendricks, Gay, 184, 185
history: future and, 116–18
  personal, 115
  rewiring, 13
Hof, Wim, 171
home, x, 88
  help with, 151
  master of, 31–33, 176, 212
  movement at, 109
  redesigning, 124
hormones, xiii, xiv, 142
  imbalances, 94
  sex, 111
  stress, 141, 142
Hubbard, Barbara Marx, 17
hunger, 52, 67, 93, 99–102

identity, 5, 17, 137, 165, 186, 189
  digesting, 81–82
  emerging, 38, 72

past, 73, 81–82, 83, 89, 167
shape-shifting, 46, 83
space and, 72–79
identity evolution, 5, 11, 42, 46–49,
    52, 71, 153, 156, 167, 179, 213
  cycle, 164, 164 (fig.)
immune function, xiv, 94, 100, 110,
    111, 142
Impact-Effort-Grid, 168 (fig.), 169,
    178, 179, 214
  excavating ease with, 167–68
improvements, 52, 83, 88, 98, 113, 169
  continuous, 112
  self-, 72, 80
inflammation, 94, 142, 171
  chronic, 103, 111
inhaling, 91, 95, 102, 143, 173
integrity, xiii, xx, 25, 42, 162, 182
  gaps in, 163, 167
  mastering, 38, 214
intelligence, 28, 45, 54, 65
  cellular, 52
  unique, 61
intuition, xvi, xx, 24, 38, 47, 88, 109,
    183
  communicating by, 96
  regret and, 14
  trusting, 60
ishvara pranidhana, xvi
  defined, 204

James, William, 159
Janet, Pierre, 159
Jarvis, Paul, 120, 178
journaling, xv, 8, 10, 11, 21, 58, 112, 117
journey, 118
  growth, 166
  healing, 166
  phases of, 54
journey map, ten-year, 53–54
Jung, Carl, 159

kaizen, 112, 114
  defined, 204
kapha, 29, 77, 113, 143, 147
  defined, 204
karma, xv, 127, 183
  defined, 204

space element, xiii, xiv, 25, 31, 35, 45,
    176, 179
    accessing, 28
    air element and, 139
    assessing, 33–34
    clutter-free, xvii, 73
    energy from, 24
    expansion and, 82–83, 139
    focus on, xxi
    mastering, 34, 182
    noticing, 28
    power of, xiv, 25
    reengineering, 182
    resources for, 207
    upgrading, 213
spanda, 99, 144, 165, 172
    defined, 205
    healthy, 166 (fig.)
spirit, 23, 24, 38, 70, 82, 109, 146
    deep quiet of, 50
    illumination of, 136
    messages for, 96
    nurturing, 89
    supporting, 144
spiritual, 23, 93, 99, 183
spiritual practices, 6, 28, 79, 144, 147,
    184
stability, 91, 101, 177
    qualities of, 25
sthira, 85, 86, 87, 88, 156
    defined, 205
stillness, 28, 85, 88, 156
Stone, Michael, 84–85
stories: fuel from, 116–18
    writing, 117, 119
Strategic Coach, 38, 147, 184
strategies, 118, 127, 128, 132, 136,
    137, 148
    action plans and, 131
    building, xviii, 36, 119, 126, 127,
        129–31
    critical issues and, 129–31
    time for, 123
strengths, xviii, xx, 12, 33, 118, 124,
    127, 129, 130
    communicating, 62
    described, 125
    developing, 62, 154
    finding, 61, 62
    immune, 34

key, 128
leveraging, 43, 61–63
physical, 106
reflecting on, 67
stress, xiii, xiv, xviii, 74, 88, 96, 148
    compounding, 140
    cycle, 101
    levels, 141
Stress in America, online survey by,
    140–41
stretching, 108, 109, 110, 112
Students Concerned About Tomorrow
    (SCAT), xi
stuff: communal, 80
    freeing space of, 88
    keeping, 84
    personal, 80
    sorting, 80, 89
sukha, 74, 85, 86, 88
    defined, 205
Sullivan, Dan, 38, 147, 148, 184
SuperAger, 78
superheroine, 57, 71, 80, 122
    journey of, 46, 47, 48, 49
    qualities of, 76–77
    sorting by, 77–79
    traction for, 74
Superheroine Infographic, 46–49, 47
    (fig.), 212
support, 154, 155, 170–73
    goals and, xix
svadyaya, xx
svastha, 73, 88
    defined, 205
svatantrya, 18
    defined, 206
Svoboda, Robert, 94, 127
SWOT, 124–27, 128, 129, 133, 136
synergy, 129, 184

tai chi, 50
Tao, 93
Tao Te Ching, 159
Taoism, 93
tapas, 116, 120, 183
    defined, 206
tarpaka kapha, 9, 14
    defined, 206

technology, 10, 49, 58, 85, 177

tejas, 116, 123, 131, 136
   defined, 206

Tesla, Nikola, 73

testing small, 43, 54–56, 153
   learning big and, 56
   thinking big and, 56, 94, 148, 171

thinking, 170
   awareness of, 143
   clear, 153
   critical, 14
   design, 54, 153
   difficult, 123, 131
   habitual, 19
   liminal, 8, 19, 121, 122, 145
   movement versus, 94
   out-of-the-box, 140
   rational, 23
   startup-and-design, 54

thinking big, 43, 54–56, 59, 120
   testing small and, 56, 94, 148, 171

3rd Alternative: Solving Life's Most Difficult Problems, The (Covey), 184

thoughts, xi, 38, 46, 50, 72, 74, 96, 141, 186
   capturing, 121
   controlling, 142
   space and, 72–79, 142

threats, 125, 130
   described, 126

three-year vision, 118, 126, 128, 130, 136, 159, 168, 182
   achieving, 157, 179
   capacities for, 162
   desires and, 178
   developing, 119, 124, 125, 129, 163, 164
   needs of, 137
   quest for, 119–23
   reading, 125, 145
   roots of, 133 (fig.)
   sharing, 213

thriving, 42, 81, 97
   orientation for, 43–44

time, x, xiii, xiv, 15, 140, 159, 176
   blocks of, 21, 151, 157
   buffer, 157
   evolution and, 153
   focus, 157
   growing, 151

   mastering, 17, 36, 136, 140, 141, 145, 156, 157, 213–14
   possibilities regarding, 142
   progress and, 152
   shape-shifting, 139, 141
   as spiritual practice, 148
   winds of, 156

time-frame, 154, 176

tools, 48, 56, 117
   developing, xvi
   family-related, xv
   project-management, 136, 152

transformation, x, xi, xx, 5, 14, 18, 24, 105, 120, 159
   friction for, 26
   guiding, xv–xvi
   metabolic force of, 29
   seasonal, 136

triadic forces, 30 (fig.)

triggers, 13, 15, 21, 87, 88

Triggers: Becoming the Person You Want to Be (Goldsmith), 12–13

12 Rules of Life (Peterson), 117

12 Week Year, The (Moran), 127, 148

underworld, 164, 165
   mapping, 162–63, 214

Upper Limit Problem, 184

US Army War College, 42

US Centers for Disease Control (CDC), 110

vairagya, 75, 83
   defined, 206

values, xvi, xix, 5, 41, 59, 72, 154, 177, 212
   adding, 89, 179
   code of, 81
   common, 72, 79–81
   possessions and, 34
   shared, 80, 81
   space and, 34

vata, 29, 77, 112, 144, 147
   defined, 206

vayu, 139
   defined, 206

vibration, 73–77, 78, 79, 82, 85, 88
   positive, 186
   space and, 73, 74

vision, x, xiv, xviii, 73, 118, 145, 161
    actions and, 136
    commitment to, 129
    critical, 36
    future and, 119mapping, 121
    pursuing, 124, 137, 182
    reflecting, 14
    See also three-year vision
vision-planning, 15, 118, 155, 174,
        176
viveka, 75, 77, 83
    defined, 206
voice, 14, 16, 21
    inner, 8
    power of, 66
volatile, uncertain, complex, ambiguous
        (VUCA), 42, 44

waking, 93, 143, 152, 188
water, xx, 31, 37, 160, 182
    drinking, 104
    healing, 179
    noticing, 27
water element, xiii, xxi, 32, 45, 156,
        176, 214
    accepting, 178
    activating, 183
    assessing, 37–38
    energy from, 24
    intelligence of, 26
    mastering, 38, 159, 160, 178
    power of, xiv, 38, 162
    resources for, 208
    wisdom of, 164–67
weaknesses, 12, 118, 124, 125, 128,
        130, 174
    critical, 126, 129
    described, 126
wealth, xvi, 54
    dynamics, 61, 62
Wheeler, Kristen, 61
willingness, 22
    displaying, 17
    readiness versus, 16–17
Willink, Jocko, 152
Willpower Doesn't Work (Hardy), 72
wisdom, ix, 11, 18, 27, 31, 50, 65, 118,
        164, 167, 172, 179, 181, 189
    ancient, xi, xii
    inner, xiii, 24

intrinsic, 25
intuitive, xxi, 24
universal, 27
work, 16, 42, 155
    flows, 186
    movement at, 109
workouts, 35, 56, 93, 107, 114

yearning, 9, 11
    digesting, 13–14
    empowering, 10
    mining, 119
    regret and, 12
    voices of, 14, 16, 21
yoga, xi, xiii, 5, 6, 19, 24, 31, 39, 50,
        75, 91, 93, 100, 105, 112, 151,
        172, 173
    defined, 206
    resources for, 208
Yogahealer.com, xi, xii, xiv, 151, 153
yogis, 6, 18, 19, 51, 82, 116, 141, 142,
        171, 183

BOOK CLUB IDEAS

hen *Master of You* becomes a conversation about taking action, you can get traction. Forming a book club with a friend or two, in person or online, makes all the difference. The Master of You format lends itself to women's career groups, to yoga studios, and to personal growth–oriented book clubs.

The best way is for a book club to dive into the book and workbook over six months. Form accountability partners to check in weekly and reinforce taking the actions and doing the exercises.

Month 1: Do the exercises in part 1.

Month 2: Do the exercises in
chapter 4, "Space: Master of Home."

Month 3: Do the exercises in
chapter 5, "Earth: Master of Body."

Month 4: Do the exercises in
chapter 6, "Fire: Master of Ambition."

Month 5: Do the exercises in
chapter 7, "Air: Master of Time."

Month 6: Do the exercises in
chapter 8, "Water: Master of Integrity and Flow."

Below are some suggested questions to help guide and start off the discussion each month. Use the strategies in this chapter to troubleshoot past any difficulties in working through the habits.

The workbook that accompanies the book is free to everyone in your group, available at masterofyou.us/workbook. Have your group members print the workbook, put it in a binder, and bring it to your meet-ups!

To reinforce taking action and sharing results, which will help you inspire each other, create a group on a social platform, such as a free private Facebook group.

MONTH 1   PART 1

- Find your why . . . for doing the rest of the book.
  Take notes to remind each other down the road.

  - "I can't wait until _____."

  - "Who I'd like to become next is _____."

  - "The next purpose hidden at the very
    root of my self may be _____."

- Discuss the Master of You ethos. What is appealing? What would be challenging for you to live as your values?

- Share your Superheroine Infographic.

- Share your Native Strengths and personality profiles.

MONTH 2   SPACE: MASTER OF HOME

- Start the meeting with the breathing
  exercise Expand Your Inner Space.

- Explain why you chose your five words.

- Describe how those words support your constitution or your next identity evolution.

- What emotions are arising as you sort your stuff? What identities are being digested?

- How is upgrading your space affecting your ability to focus and rejuvenate?

MONTH 3   EARTH: MASTER OF BODY

- Start the meeting with the Five-Bodies Check-in.

- Share which of the three body rhythms needs your attention. What does aiming for a solid B– in this body rhythm look like?

- Discuss what worked in your one-week experiment.

MONTH 4   FIRE: MASTER OF AMBITION

- Share what emerged in writing your story.

- Share your three-year vision. Coach each other to be specific so you'll know when you have arrived.

- Share your critical issues.

- Share your one-year milestones.

MONTH 5   AIR: MASTER OF TIME

- Share your ideal calendar.

- Share your chief findings and where you can take immediate action on what you no longer want to do. Help each other find qualified people.

- If you've started alignment meetings (with yourself or your people), what is working? When is a good time to do alignment meetings with yourself for your seasonal milestones?

MONTH 6   WATER: MASTER OF INTEGRITY AND FLOW

- What did you discover in mapping your underworld? You can revisit any of the questions from that exercise for a discussion.

- When you look back at the biggest breakthroughs or achievements of your life, what were the breakdowns that led to the breakthroughs?

- In the Impact-Effort Grid exercise, what are your highest-impact, lowest-effort actions to test next? What are your high-effort, but necessary for high impact, efforts you should put into your seasonal milestones?

- What self-compassionate activities—such as hot baths or cold plunges—will support you in your identity evolution this month?

CONCLUSION   WHO ARE YOU BECOMING?

- Start by doing the Recalibration Practice together.

- Share how you are expanding beyond your upper limit.

- Discuss how you are becoming a leader of us as you become a master of you. Where is this showing up in your life?

- Strengthen your group by deciding if you want to go another round together over the next six months, reiterating and mastering the elements as you become a master of you.

ABOUT THE AUTHOR

Cate Stillman has been innovating practical, experiential, evolutionary courses using the wisdom tradition of Ayurveda and yoga since founding Yogahealer.com in 2001. Her first book, *Body Thrive: Uplevel Your Body and Your Life with the 10 Habits of Ayurveda and Yoga*, emerged from teaching local and global online communities and supports her Yoga Health Coaching organization, Yogahealer.com, spreading thrive around the planet.

Master of You evolved from years of experimentation with her online community. The best way to access Cate and the global Yogahealer.com community is to listen to her podcast, the Yogahealer Real Life Show, join her email list to receive the many free resources, or attend a Yogahealer live event.

Cate and her husband are raising their child in Alta, Wyoming, to ski and mountain bike and in Punta Mita, Mexico, to surf and be bicultural. Her cat, Dukkha, practiced vairagyam by sleeping through the creation of this book.

ABOUT SOUNDS TRUE

Sounds True is a multimedia publisher whose mission is to inspire and support personal transformation and spiritual awakening. Founded in 1985 and located in Boulder, Colorado, we work with many of the leading spiritual teachers, thinkers, healers, and visionary artists of our time. We strive with every title to preserve the essential "living wisdom" of the author or artist. It is our goal to create products that not only provide information to a reader or listener but also embody the quality of a wisdom transmission.

For those seeking genuine transformation, Sounds True is your trusted partner. At SoundsTrue.com you will find a wealth of free resources to support your journey, including exclusive weekly audio interviews, free downloads, interactive learning tools, and other special savings on all our titles.

To learn more, please visit SoundsTrue.com/freegifts or call us toll-free at 800.333.9185.

In loving memory of Beth Skelley, book designer extraordinaire. Her spirit lives on in our books and in our hearts.

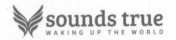